The
New Normal

Also by Jennifer Ashton, M.D., M.S.

The Body Scoop for Girls
Your Body Beautiful
Eat This, Not That! When You're Expecting
Life After Suicide
The Self-Care Solution

The
New Normal

A ROADMAP
TO RESILIENCE IN
THE PANDEMIC ERA

Jennifer Ashton, M.D., M.S.

with Sarah Toland

WM

WILLIAM MORROW

An Imprint of HarperCollinsPublishers

This book contains advice and information relating to healthcare. It is not intended to replace medical advice and should be used to supplement rather than replace regular care by your doctor. It is recommended that you seek your physician's advice before embarking on any medical program or treatment. All efforts have been made to assure the accuracy of the information contained in this book as of the date of publication. The publisher and the author disclaim liability for any medical outcomes that may occur as a result of applying the methods suggested in this book.

THE NEW NORMAL. Copyright © 2021 by JLA Enterprises Corporation. All rights reserved. Printed in the United States of America. No part of this book may be used or reproduced in any manner whatsoever without written permission except in the case of brief quotations embodied in critical articles and reviews. For information, address HarperCollins Publishers, 195 Broadway, New York, NY 10007.

HarperCollins books may be purchased for educational, business, or sales promotional use. For information, please email the Special Markets Department at SPsales@harpercollins.com.

FIRST EDITION

Library of Congress Cataloging-in-Publication Data has been applied for.

ISBN 978-0-06-308323-3

21 22 23 24 25 LSC 10 9 8 7 6 5 4 3 2 1

To all the essential workers, to everyone who has been personally affected by COVID-19, directly or indirectly, and to everyone everywhere working toward the prevention and treatment of this virus . . .

And to Alex and Chloe: You continue to be my Universe.

Contents

Introduction

Several months into the coronavirus pandemic, I was running through Central Park when it suddenly struck me that everything was different. Central Park looked largely the same—it's one of the few immutable aspects in a city that never sleeps. But the people in the park were different—everyone in masks, far more joggers, and far fewer tourists. Then there was me: I was actually running in the park, which wasn't typical. But since I don't go to the gym anymore, running outside has become my new normal.

Just as I was finishing my new workout, I nearly ran into several dozen people standing on the sidewalk at the end of the park. This was odd: New Yorkers don't just stand idly on the street. This is a city that moves and moves quickly, but it now appeared that people seemed to have fewer places to go or less incentive to go anywhere in a rush.

Then I realized what they were doing: They were standing in line to go inside a Whole Foods Market nearby. The line snaked around the block, with people standing six feet apart on bright green decals plastered on the pavement. Every time a shopper exited the store, a security guard let someone in, reminding them to follow the one-way aisle arrows around the store.

This was hardly an unusual sight. Lines were forming outside stores all over the city and across the country. But it wasn't until that moment that I realized what it meant: If everyday activities like how we exercise and shop for food have changed so significantly, nothing in our world will ever be the same again, even if or when we find a cure for COVID-19. The coronavirus crisis has been like an asteroid hitting Earth: Our world has been permanently impacted and indelibly reshaped. It was like someone had suddenly unfurled a big banner across the end of Central Park that read WELCOME TO THE NEW WORLD. Everything here is different. Take a good look around. And get used to it.

Months later, the new world that I first witnessed outside Central Park is now our new normal. Lines at grocery stores have come and gone and regulations have inevitably changed, but the endpoint is the same: The asteroid has hit, and it's ushered in a whole new era. And in the pandemic era, what we do, how we think, what we fear, and what we believe in are all drastically different and will be for years to come.

I've never seen anything like it before—no one has. The coronavirus pandemic is the greatest single story of our lifetime. Nothing in my career as a doctor or medical correspondent has even remotely approached the COVID-19 narrative in terms of its social, medical, economic, political, physical, mental, and emotional fallout. During this fallout, I've had a front-row seat, watching the story unfold, interpreting its twists and turns, and then analyzing and retelling it for millions of viewers.

I've been with ABC News since 2012 and the chief medical correspondent for the network since 2017. I've appeared regularly on *Good Morning America, World News Tonight with David Muir, Nightline,* and other national programming. But when the outbreak began, I started to go on air for up to thirteen-plus hours per day and started broadcasting the show *GMA3: What You Need to Know* with Amy Robach. Since then, I've lived, slept, and even dreamed COVID-19, reading all the research and speaking regularly with epidemiology experts, public health officials, infectious disease specialists, and Dr. Anthony Fauci, the country's top infectious disease doctor. I've been to the CDC headquarters in Atlanta; the United States' vaccine development lab in Bethesda, Maryland; and the West Wing of the White House.

Through it all, I've been left with one major takeaway: We will never be the same again. Not you, not me, not your next-door neighbor, not the guy or gal halfway around the world. If you lived through 9/11, you know what a crisis can do to a country. September 11 opened our eyes to a previously inconceivable threat and permanently changed the lives of thousands of Americans, along with how we travel, what we fear, and the economic, political, social, and physical landscape of the biggest city in the United States.

The pandemic has not only altered our everyday activities like where we exercise and how we shop but also upended basic human necessities like how we eat, sleep, work, and interact with others. What was normal about being in an office, going out to eat, or seeing friends and family in 2019 isn't today. Just like 9/11, the pandemic has also opened our eyes to a new, previously inconceivable threat—a never-before-seen, high-impact respiratory pathogen—and transformed how we approach our health, what we perceive is important, and even what we perceive is possible.

If you've flown on a plane in the last twenty years, you know that travel never went back to "normal" after 9/11. Similarly, the world won't ever go back to what life was like B.C. (before coronavirus), even if we develop an effective vaccine and treatment protocol. When I hear people say "when things go back to normal," my heart pains a bit: Things aren't going back to normal because this *is* our new normal. That's a really important concept to understand.

As a doctor, I can say with assurance the coronavirus isn't going anywhere anytime soon. Infectious illnesses like COVID-19 that are highly transmissible but not consistently deadly are the hardest to control, while diseases like Ebola that are more lethal but also more difficult to contract are generally easier to contain and eradicate. For proof, just look at the flu, which is highly transmissible and not as deadly—and something doctors are still trying to get under control.

Instead of waiting for science to outsmart the virus—because we could be waiting a long time if the flu and common cold are any indicators—we have to figure out how to live with the virus and manage it so it doesn't manage us. We'll need different degrees of management at different times, of course, but this is our new normal. There likely won't be a point in your lifetime when you will be able to say *corona-what*?

There's another reason our "old normal" is never coming back. Even if we attain herd immunity or find a cure for COVID-19, it's likely the planet will face another viral outbreak of the same proportions, if not even worse than COVID-19. Emerging infectious disease specialists tell us that another pandemic isn't a matter of *if*, but *when*. We now know this can happen because we've seen it happen. The latent threat of another pandemic has significant psychological implications and will impact the world in many ways, including some that are unforeseen to us right now.

What you can expect, however, is for people to think twice for years to come about being inside crowded spaces. Many won't be eager to hug, and the handshake, as Dr. Fauci already declared, is likely dead. Hand-sanitizing stations aren't going to disappear from public places anytime soon. Some people will continue to wear masks inside public areas for the rest of their lives. Almost all of us will think at every cough or sneeze, *Be careful, wash your hands, stay at least six feet away, don't touch your face.*

If this sounds a little like post-traumatic stress disorder (PTSD), that's because it is: The pandemic has been tragic, terrifying, and disruptive enough that all of us have a touch of PTSD in the new normal. The next time you hear about a bad flu strain or a new viral outbreak, you'll likely cringe and prepare for the worst. You may have flashbacks to when lockdown orders were initiated across the country at the beginning of the outbreak or feel a sense of deep foreboding, dread, or even depression.

While this is our new normal, it's not a reality that has to be frightening—or even unfamiliar—and that's exactly why I wrote this book. My goal is to help you recognize and adapt to our new normal, because the sooner and more seamlessly you do, the sooner our new normal won't be new anymore, but just normal. I want to help you see that we have to acknowledge that everything is different now, because only by acknowledging this can we begin to accept and heal. This is, after all, the definition of resiliency: our ability to recover readily from adversity. The more resilient you can become—physically, mentally, and emotionally—the better able you'll be to withstand any adversity, whether it's another pandemic or a personal challenge, and see it as an opportunity rather than an alarming event.

But how do you begin to find resiliency in the new normal when it feels like the rules, expectations, and risks are constantly changing? New studies contradict things that were conveyed as truth just weeks prior, while friends and family seem to have different opinions and behaviors about what constitutes actual risk. In the infodemic age—when accurate and inaccurate information is spread as rapidly as a virus itself—the amount of news and interpretations of that news is staggering. We've never had to consider so much when trying to decide whether to do something so simple as attend a friend's outdoor birthday party or go to the gym. With the stakes so high, the new normal can feel paralyzing to the point of self-isolation—or on the other hand, so overwhelming that we want to throw caution to the wind, cross our fingers, and hope for the best.

While I can understand and relate to both attitudes, I certainly don't recommend either. Instead, there's a better approach—and it starts by learning to think like a doctor. When medical decisions are complicated or involve high risk in the ER or the OR, physicians don't get paralyzed by fear or hope for the best: They act calmly, coolly, and based on the best data or science on hand.

Throughout this book, I will teach you how to think like a doctor in order to help you stay informed, make safe decisions about your health, and better navigate the new normal. You don't need an M.D. after your name to think like one—you just need to know how to take a calm, analytical, and evidence-based view of any crisis. And with this book, I'll show you exactly how.

First, though, I'm not just a doctor on TV—I'm also a real doctor who sees real patients in real life, as I've done for the last twenty years. From Day One of the pandemic, I've approached the crisis like a doctor, prioritizing evidence, not emotions. I've looked at the virus as I do a patient: What are the vital signs? What do we know about the disease? And what don't we know about the disease? But I've kept others' emotions in mind as well, as I've viewed the lens of the TV camera like the eyes of my patients: curious, frightened, and confused.

Similar to how a doctor would never diagnose you based on unknown vital signs, I've never drawn conclusions about COVID-19—or any other illness, for that matter—based on hypotheses, politics, opinion, or conjecture. As I've said on air multiple times, it's really important to say what we know *and* what we don't know. We need to rely on facts, not fear, to make the best decisions about our health in a crisis situation, just as doctors do for patients in the ER and in the OR. When you do this, you can stay calm and steady about an emotionally charged, ever-evolving situation.

What's more, a good doctor doesn't just focus on one body part or a single symptom: We look at the entire patient and the interaction of different systems to effectively diagnose and treat. Similarly, I've always taken a big-picture perspective of this pandemic. And I've passed that perspective on to viewers so they can understand what's going on without getting bogged down in specifics that can change on a day-to-day basis.

This last caveat is super important: If we've learned anything from this pandemic, it's that details of a disease can change on a dime. That's why it's critical to learn how to think like a doctor and take a big-picture perspective. It's also vital to understand how science works.

In medicine and science, doctors learn new things every day, no matter how long or intensely they've studied a specific illness or disease. A doctor can spend his or her entire lifetime researching a virus or other pathogen and still not come close to knowing everything about it. We're still learning new things about the flu, for example, even though influenza-like illnesses have been around for hundreds of years.

In the instance of a brand-new pathogen like this novel strain of the coronavirus, we haven't even begun to scratch the surface of what there is to know. That's why I think it's vital that we focus on what we know *now*, which means what medicine and science have shown us to date, while also incorporating what we know about other coronaviruses to help inform our analysis. New risk factors for COVID-19 could always emerge and the virus could change, which means medical information and advice should change with it.

At the same time, it's important to trust the facts we have at hand: evidence over emotion, medicine over make-believe, and science over sham. No virus in the history of humankind has been studied so rapidly and intensely as the coronavirus, and the amount of knowledge we've amassed in a short period of time is breathtaking, impressive, and reassuring.

I'm not tone deaf, though. I know there's more mistrust about medicine and the media right now than ever. If you're skeptical, cynical, or scared, that's okay, understandable, and actually appropriate. I'll be the first to admit I don't have all the answers—no one does. And the thing is, no one ever will—which is why it's never about having all the answers in the first place and instead about knowing the right questions to ask. If you can learn to do this, you'll be able to get the information you need to better navigate our new normal or any challenging crisis you might find yourself in.

I want to recognize, too, that everyone's situation is unique. Maybe you lost a family member, friend, or colleague to COVID-19—that's a tragic reality to face. Or maybe you lost your job, your home, or your business in the pandemic. My heart goes out to you. Or perhaps you got sick with COVID-19 and are still recovering. Maybe you're figuring out how to work from home permanently and/or are juggling children or older relatives in your household 24/7. Or maybe you're an essential worker who's never had the luxury of working from home this entire time. No matter your new normal, my goal is to help you navigate it. You can read this book start to finish or cherry-pick the parts that to appeal you, but I promise everyone can find something in every chapter.

Whether it's prioritizing the urgency of our own health, learning how to decipher complicated medical news, or simply understanding how to make what we eat and how we sleep work better for our bodies in stressful times, there are takeaways from the pandemic that can lead us all to healthier, happier lives. The coronavirus outbreak has been brutal, but the changes it's inspired don't have to be. Our new normal is a different place, to be sure, but it can also be a good one. And if you follow the roadmap to resilience that you'll find inside this book, you'll discover many hidden gems inherent in the coronavirus crisis along the way.

One of the biggest gems, in my opinion, is that the pandemic has given us all a stronger sense of solidarity. Today, it's not just one person adapting to our new normal—it's all of us. Every single person has lost something in the pandemic, whether it was a family member, friend, business, job, their health, or their freedom. Some of us may have lost something less crucial, like our ability to go to the gym, eat at restaurants, travel, or see family and friends with abandon, but we still lost something. This means we're all grieving together—and getting over it together. The human spirit has never been stronger.

One of the greatest gifts of the pandemic, if you can find it and choose to accept it, is gratitude. It can be difficult, but I want to remind you with this book that we have a choice: We can either dwell on what we've lost or remind ourselves of all the things we still have. Even more important, we can choose to see what we've gained through adversity. And I promise you that we've all gained something.

Finally, while everything is different in our new normal, there are two things that haven't changed: laughter and love. I take a lot of strength from this fact. Laughter and love have never disappeared in times of war, peace, pandemics, or great health and prosperity. No matter what happens in our world next, you can always find laughter and love. And choosing to look for both—now and always—will serve as your GPS on the ultimate road to resiliency.

CHAPTER 1

Body

It happened on a public bus in Detroit.

A woman coughed repetitively. She didn't cover her mouth. She didn't seem to have any concern for others.

Jason Hargrove was driving that bus in March 2020. He was so angered by the incident that afterward he posted an eight-minute-long video on Facebook about what happened, pleading with people to take seriously what we were calling the novel coronavirus.

Eleven days later, Jason was dead from COVID-19. The fifty-year-old father of six died alone in the hospital, without his wife or any of his children by his side.

Days later, his widow, Desha Johnson Hargrove, appeared on *Good Morning America* to share his story, which had already made headlines around the world. Speaking exclusively with correspondent T. J. Holmes, she begged people to stay at home and take the recommended precautions so that her husband's death wouldn't be in vain.

Months later, Desha told me that she still felt people weren't taking the pandemic seriously. "This is not a norm that anyone thought we'd see, but this is where we are," she told me by phone. "And I want to help anyone from being in the spot that I am right now."

Desha is right. This is not a norm any of us ever thought we'd see. It's a *new* normal. But we now know a lot more than we did in March 2020. And we know that there are specific, impactful steps we can take to avoid ending up in the same spot Desha has found herself in: severely impacted by COVID-19. We can take precautions like wearing masks and physically distancing to help prevent others from getting seriously ill or dying from the disease. We can also take precautions that go way beyond wearing a cloth face covering to keep ourselves from getting very ill.

From a doctor's perspective, I know that Jason had several risk factors that made him more vulnerable to serious illness with COVID-19. He was a black man, and we now know that people of color and men, in general, are more likely to develop severe complications from the virus. He also worked an essential job that put him at risk during the height of the early outbreak.

While Jason couldn't change his gender or his color, he had other risk factors that we have since learned likely made him more vulnerable to the virus. Desha told me that her husband was overweight and diabetic and had high blood pressure—three of the biggest predictors of serious COVID-19 complications that people *can* potentially change. By the time researchers discovered this about the virus, it was too late for Jason. But it's not too late for everyone else.

"This virus is taking no prisoners," she told me. "And if you have these underlying issues, you could be affected. People who are obese—we can manage that. We can take control of that."

Desha told me she is also overweight and now doing everything she can to make sure her story doesn't end like her husband's did. "Get out there and go for a walk. Drink your water. Eat healthier," she told me. "And I'm talking to me, Desha, because I don't want to be another Jason story. I can't just give a message—I have *to be* the message."

Desha's story is powerful. It's also all too common. The majority of coronavirus patients featured on *Good Morning America* have been overweight or obese. Many have suffered from diabetes, high blood pressure, or other chronic conditions. Similarly, the majority of those whom I've known personally who've been hospitalized or died from the disease were black, overweight or obese, and/or had underlying conditions.

It's a difficult truth to face, but as more time has passed, and living with the virus has become our new way of life, we have a clearer understanding of the preexisting health issues that are most available to exploitation by the virus. Now that we know what will make us more susceptible to the virus, it's up to us to do something about it and try everything in our power to get these conditions under control. Health risks like diabetes and obesity don't mean the same things that they used to—now they are much more concerning. Jason didn't have a choice—the science didn't exist when he became infected. But you do, and now's the time to be proactive about your health and your ability to survive and thrive in the world's new normal.

One of the most critical lessons I've learned after almost a year of reporting daily on national TV about COVID-19 is this: Doing everything you can to be as healthy as you can possibly be right now is one of the best ways to pandemic-proof your body and adapt physically to the additional health risks that COVID-19 carries. As a practicing doctor for the past twenty years, I know that every single person on the planet, you included, has ways and means of mitigating disease risk, whether we're talking about cancer, coronavirus, or some other microorganism that makes up the world's next pandemic. I don't need to know everything about a specific pathogen or your individual medical history per se to know ways in which to help you minimize the negative effects of disease.

That said, after incessant reading of the top studies conducted on the coronavirus to date, talking with the world's top infectious disease specialists, and distilling what I find to millions of ABC News viewers almost daily, I know that there are specific conditions that make us much more vulnerable to COVID-19—and specific steps we can take to significantly reduce our risk.

If you've been lucky enough to avoid the virus so far, that's fantastic. But if we've learned anything since New Year's Eve of 2019, when the first case of COVID-19 was identified in Wuhan, China, it's that the coronavirus works in mysterious ways, striking in widely disparate degrees of severity at any time, no matter who are you, where you live, or how much money you make.

I often use analogies on air when I talk about healthcare because medicine is complicated. So here are some others ways to look at it. Let's say that, in one or two months' time, you're asked to do something that will take all your energy, like run an Olympic race, give a high-stakes presentation at work, or take a final exam. If you know that you'll be put to the test in this way, would you start doing everything now to prepare? Or would you wait until you were toeing the starting line, standing in front of your entire office, or sitting down for the test to start getting ready?

Preparation is the name of the game in pandemic times, as we have no idea if and when we could get infected and how severely we might react. While doctors like me have been warning people for years that we should focus on our overall health and weight, the need has never been more urgent. I know you've heard before—likely many times over the years—how important it is to prioritize your health and take better care of yourself, but that advice means something different today than it did in 2019. We have to do everything possible now—train for that race, prepare for the presentation, study for the final—in order to improve our chances of not only performing our best but also crushing it, if and when our day ever comes.

Consider this is your wake-up call. It's time to train and to help pandemic-proof your body as much as possible, and I'm here to show you how.

WEIGHT LOSS

Where to start? The single most effective thing you can do to help pandemic-proof your body is to lose weight. That's because being overweight or obese is the biggest chronic risk factor to developing severe COVID-19 complications. Obesity is a bigger risk factor than cancer, heart disease, and other serious illnesses. It's even a bigger risk factor than respiratory conditions like asthma, emphysema, and lung disease.

Here are the facts: In August 2020, a meta-analysis that included nearly 400,000 patients found that those who were obese and contracted COVID-19 were 113 percent more likely than people of healthy weight to be hospitalized, 78 percent more likely to be admitted to the ICU, and 48 percent more likely to die.[1] Similarly, an April 2020 study conducted on 4,100 people with COVID-19 in New York City found that obesity was the primary predictor after age of whether someone would get seriously sick from the virus.[2] Young people who were obese were also much more likely to be hospitalized with COVID-19, even if they had no other risk factors.[3] Subsequent studies have reached the same conclusion, over and over again.

But what is it about obesity that's so incendiary for the virus? The truth is, carrying too much weight is a chronic disease state in and of itself, as qualified by the American Board of Obesity Medicine. What this means is that being overweight or obese acts like most other diseases in the body, increasing inflammation, weakening the immune system, and thwarting the body's ability to fight infection. That's all bad news for you if you happen to contract coronavirus, which menaces the body by also driving up inflammation. When you add more inflammation onto chronic inflammation, the body can't take it—it simply starts to shut down.

Compounding this issue is that, if the scales aren't tipping in your favor, you're more likely to have or to develop type 2 diabetes, high blood pressure, and heart disease, all of which also put you at a much greater risk for severe illness or death from COVID-19.

This is not good news for most people, I understand. Two-thirds of all Americans are overweight or obese. The condition is so widespread, in fact, that if you are overweight, you may think you're perfectly healthy because everyone around you looks the same. Some of my patients fall into this mindset, and it's a real problem. Because if you don't realize that you're walking around with a potentially deadly disease, you're likely not taking all the precautions you need to now.

I want to make something crystal clear about obesity, however: If you are overweight or obese, you are not to blame. Obesity is not a disease brought on by laziness or lack of discipline. There are genetic, metabolic, nutritional, hormonal, and behavioral components to the condition, along with many other complex factors. Sometimes prescription medication alone can cause excess weight gain. I've seen so many of my own patients struggle with this, and I know how difficult the issue can be. And I'm here to help. I know it may seem like a futile effort or an uphill battle. I know the "I've tried it all, and nothing works" history of many with the conditions of obesity or overweight. This is not a character flaw—it's a medical condition, and now is the time to address it as such, without judgment, blame, or shame.

Being overweight or obese isn't your fault. But no matter what your experience has been like in the past, I want to help you try to continue to make strides to change your situation—now more than ever before, because your life may depend on it. And if you haven't paid attention to your weight, nutrition, or fitness levels before, now is also the time to start doing something about it—STAT.

Weight loss isn't easy—if it were, there wouldn't be a multi-billion-dollar diet industry built around helping people drop anywhere from three to three hundred pounds. But losing weight to lower your risks from COVID-19 is unlike any kind of weight loss you've tried. That's because dropping pounds for a pandemic isn't the same as getting ready for summer swimsuit season. You don't need to be a size 2 or look like a model to survive and thrive in our new normal. The goal shouldn't be huge, dramatic, and unattainable weight loss. Instead, it should be to get your BMI in a healthy range. If you're motivated to lose more—especially once you get started and realize how good losing weight can feel—that's a bonus that will only strengthen your physical and mental arsenal.

Here are ten steps to take to help pandemic-proof your body:

1. **Assess whether your weight is a problem.** If you think you may be overweight or obese, you probably are. In our heart of hearts, most of us know whether our weight is a health problem. To be sure though, go online and calculate your body mass index (BMI)—the measurement and accompanying scale will indicate if you're overweight or obese. Your BMI isn't a perfect assessment by any means—muscle weighs more than fat, which is why some athletes have immoderately high BMIs. But the measurement has been clinically correlated to specific health outcomes hundreds of times, and it's one of the best free, readily available measurements we have.

   If you'd feel better with a medical diagnosis that you're overweight or obese, make an appointment with an obesity-medicine physician, your primary-care doctor, or a healthcare provider. You may want to see a doctor at this time anyway, especially if you haven't been to one in more than a year (learn more about a pandemic physical on page 29).

2. **Drop the blame game.** If you are overweight or obese, remind yourself that it's not your fault and that you didn't do anything wrong. Allowing yourself to wallow in guilt can make it more difficult to adopt the mindset you need to lose weight.

3. **Be willing to try and tell yourself you CAN.** It's just like the story of *The Little Engine That Could:* If you think you can't lose weight, you probably won't. Lots of people stay stuck at an unhealthy weight because they've already accepted that they can't lose it. Don't be one of those people. Every one of us is capable of amazing things. Choose to be the little engine that could and believe in yourself.

4. **Put a carrot at the end of the stick.** Not a real carrot, of course, but rewarding yourself with a non-food item when you lose a certain amount of weight can help motivate you to stay the course. Promise to treat yourself to a new pair of shoes, for example, or a day out with friends, or another material item or special experience if you drop ten pounds. Set similar incentives for twenty, thirty, forty pounds, etc., depending on how much you have to lose.

5. **Pick a weight-loss plan from this doctor-approved device.** One of the simplest strategies for weight loss and weight management comes from a lecture I attended while becoming board certified in obesity medicine: a three-tiered obesity-treatment pyramid that boils weight loss down to three distinct action plans.[4] If you're overweight, with a BMI equal to or greater than 25—or even if you're at an ideal weight—choose the bottom tier of the pyramid, which prescribes healthy nutrition and exercise (see steps 6–8), or what I like to refer to as the Two F's: Food and Fitness. The middle tier advocates FDA-approved weight-loss medications, which an obesity-medicine specialist or other licensed provider can prescribe to

those who are clinically obese, with a BMI equal to or greater than 30. The top tier of the pyramid recommends bariatric surgery, like sleeve gastrectomy, for those with a BMI equal to or greater than 40, which qualifies as extremely obese and is life-threatening.

6. **Stop agonizing over what you eat.** Most people don't lose weight because they follow restrictive diets or crazy food fads. The truth is, you don't have to cut out multiple food groups, eat only green vegetables, or count calories or carbs for months or years on end—oftentimes, these types of diets can be effective in the short term, but they're almost never sustainable. Instead, focus on eating until you're satisfied, not stuffed, and on consuming less food throughout the day.

7. **Prioritize low-sugar and low-carb consumption.** We'll go into detail about the best nutrition for our new normal in chapter 4, but prioritizing foods high in protein and healthy fat and low in sugar and carbohydrates is the most effective way to lose weight. You don't have to start counting carbs— instead, reduce the amount you eat so that carbs make up only a quarter of every meal. In addition, don't snack on processed foods like crackers, bread, chips, or baked goods, even if they're gluten-free or plant-based.

8. **Move more, but don't assume exercise will save you.** Ninety percent of your ability to lose weight depends on the foods you eat (or don't eat). Only 10 percent of your weight depends on how much you exercise. Moving more will certainly build muscle, improve your health, and help you lose weight faster and keep it off longer. But don't make the mistake of relying too heavily on exercise to compensate for a junk-food diet if you want to lose weight.

9. **Beware of quick fixes.** If it sounds too good to be true, it probably is. The weight-loss industry is full of quick fixes, scams,

and "cures," all of which prey on people's desperation and frustration. Despite what you may see on social media, however, very few of these fixes are actually effective, and they can be unsafe.

10. **Be patient.** Losing weight takes time. Being overweight or obese didn't happen to you overnight and it's not going to be fixed overnight.

Do You Still Need to Pandemic-Proof Your Body If You Get a Vaccine?

Yes. And here's why: It's just good health. As the pandemic has made clear, the risks of obesity and other chronic health conditions like diabetes and heart disease aren't just theoretical— they are very real and potentially very deadly. Doctors have been warning people about these conditions for years, and they'll always pose a threat with or without a pandemic. Even with a vaccine that reduces the risk of COVID-19 infection, we all still need to prioritize our health. COVID-19 has helped to show us that chronic health problems like obesity and heart disease aren't abstract, and there's no way of knowing when and what the next pandemic might bring. Get vaccinated and take every step possible to be as healthy as you can in our new normal.

BEYOND THE SCALE: OTHER RISK FACTORS

While losing weight is the most important thing you can do to lower your risk of COVID-19, there are other critical research-backed ways to bolster your health in our new normal based on what we know about the disease.

At the beginning of the pandemic, I must have said the word *comorbidities* on national television dozens of times, which is much more often than I ever did in medical school or residency. I wasn't alone, of course: The term, used to describe the presence of one or more physical complications alongside a primary health condition, was falling out of the mouth of every medical expert. In a matter of weeks, most Americans understood the pedantic term, which had previously been uttered only by doctors, medical professors, and a few characters on *Grey's Anatomy*.

For our purposes, you can think of comorbidities as the same as preexisting conditions: Both are need-to-know info in pandemic times. If a person has certain comorbidities or preexisting conditions, he or she is much more likely to be hospitalized or die from COVID-19. But not all preexisting conditions are the same. Some are riskier than others, and it's not always intuitive which ones are worse for COVID-19.

What You Can't Change

Let's start with the facts. You already know that the biggest risk factor for coronavirus is age. Older people are simply more likely to get seriously ill or die from the disease than younger people, which is why the virus has wreaked havoc on nursing homes across the country. The second biggest risk factor, as we now know, is being overweight or obese.

But after age and weight, things start to get a little murky. According to research to date, men are twice as likely to die from COVID-19 as women, despite a similar infection rate between the sexes. We have theories about why: Some comorbidities like high blood pressure (more on hypertension on page 23) and heart disease are more common among men, and women tend to have a more robust immune system than men (remember, autoimmune diseases are more common in women than in men), but no one knows for sure if this is the reason.

People of color are also much more likely to get seriously ill or die from COVID-19 than white people. This racial inequity is largely due to socioeconomic reasons. People of color are more likely to be classified low income, which means they're also more likely to have reduced access to quality healthcare, higher rates of obesity and other serious illnesses, multiple live-in family members or roommates, and jobs with greater exposure or without a work-from-home option.

The thing about risk factors such as age, gender, and race is that you can't change any of them. But knowing you're more vulnerable can help you better assess your risk tolerance for certain social activities, which we'll talk about in chapters 9 and 10. If you have a number of high-risk factors—if you're a black or brown man over age sixty-five, for example—I would encourage you to take every precaution possible, like always wearing a mask, keeping at least six feet away from others, washing your hands, and avoiding high-risk activities like eating indoors in restaurants and attending in-person religious services.

What You Can Change

After obesity, the second biggest *modifiable* risk factor for severe illness with COVID-19 is diabetes. Also known as hyperglycemia, the condition is cause for concern on its own. But when paired with COVID-19, diabetes can be deadly. People with type 2 diabetes are four times more likely to succumb to the coronavirus than those who don't have hyperglycemia, according to research.[5]

Type 2 diabetes, which often occurs in adults who gain weight, aren't active, and/or eat a standard American diet, affects more than 34 million people in the United States. The really scary part:

One in four people with the disease don't know they have it. Similarly, one-third of all Americans have prediabetes—a precursor to type 2—yet 84 percent have no idea.

Why is the combo of diabetes and COVID-19 so deadly? In basic terms, pathogens need glucose to survive—it's why bacteria and viruses grow so well in sugar-rich environments. The more glucose surging through your cells, the more a virus can replicate, spread, and cause trouble. In addition, people with diabetes tend to have a higher level of inflammation that can exacerbate COVID-19 infections, which also produce inflammation in the body. When you're diabetic and have coronavirus, it's like a kid in a toy store before Christmas: COVID-19 goes crazy.

If you know you have diabetes, now is the time to do everything possible to reverse or control the condition using a three-pronged approach of low-sugar nutrition, more exercise, and sustained weight loss. Those who have diabetes and don't know it may be at greater risk, since many are not taking the necessary precautions recommended to those most vulnerable to the virus. That's why I recommend anyone who is overweight, inactive, and/or following a standard American diet consider making an appointment for an annual physical, especially if you haven't been to the doctor in more than a year (see page 29 for more information).

Diabetes isn't the only hidden ailment for severe COVID-19 complications. High blood pressure, called the "silent killer" since it's often missed by both patients and doctors, can double your risk of dying from coronavirus.[6] If you have high blood pressure and aren't taking medication—either because you don't know you have it or aren't following proper treatment protocol—your risk of dying from COVID-19 is even greater, according to research.[7]

These stats are particularly troubling because nearly half of all Americans have high blood pressure.[8] That means approximately 50 percent of the U.S. population is in jeopardy of severe COVID-19 complications. What's more, half of those with high blood pressure—about one-quarter of the country's total population—aren't taking medication to control the condition.

Similar to the stats on diabetes and prediabetes, many people with high blood pressure don't even know they have it. High blood pressure is often asymptomatic and easily missed by doctors, especially those who don't follow the American Heart Association's testing recommendations.[9] (Learn the one thing to ask for when getting a blood pressure test on page 31.)

Why does high blood pressure increase one's risk with COVID-19? One theory is that chronic hypertension weakens blood vessels, thereby allowing the virus to more easily dock in our bodies. High blood pressure also lowers the body's immune system response.[10] Contrary to early reports, though, taking certain blood pressure medications like ACE inhibitors does *not* appear to increase the risk of severe illness with coronavirus.[11]

How do you know if you have high blood pressure? Or how can you ensure the condition is being treated properly? All the more reason to consider getting an annual physical, which we cover in depth starting on page 29.

Other risk factors for severe COVID-19 complications include cancer; serious heart conditions; heart, lung, or kidney disease; sickle cell disease; chronic obstructive pulmonary disease (COPD); and immunocompromised conditions like HIV. Other conditions like pregnancy, moderate to severe asthma, cystic fibrosis, and neurological conditions like dementia may also increase the risk of severe illness from COVID-19, but more research is needed.

THE NEW NORMAL SELF-ASSESSMENT

No matter what risks factors you have and whether they're modifiable, you can't improve what you can't measure. If you want to train your body for an Olympic event, for example, you first need to figure out where and how to start by taking a hard look at your current and past training. If you haven't run in years, have bad knees, and don't own running shoes, your training plan will look a lot different from someone who has been working out several days a week, suffers from weak calves, and has a whole closet of high-performance sneakers.

For this reason, I recommend that everyone consider taking the time to do a serious self-assessment of his or her physical and mental health right now. Given the pandemic—and the potential of another one in the future—it's really important to know what you're doing right, what you may be doing wrong, and perhaps most important, what you might be overlooking about your health that could endanger your life in our new normal.

The goal of a self-assessment is not to unearth all your flaws or make you the healthiest human on the planet. Just as with weight loss, the goal of a pandemic self-assessment is specific to our new normal. You don't have to identify every unhealthy habit you have, but focus on finding those that may increase your risk of COVID-19 and other infectious illnesses.

Consider this self-assessment to be a judgment-free zone—you just want to find possible issues so you can be aware of and fix them before they become catastrophic problems. And while everyone should strive for optimal health, your top priority now is to make sure your body can survive a health crisis—whether it's coronavirus, a bad strain of the flu, or an unknown pathogen that triggers the world's next global outbreak.

To do an honest self-assessment, you need to get your mind in the right place, too. Like most things in life, it's all about attitude and the realization that things are different now. While maybe you were able to get away with poor health habits or preexisting conditions so far, we live in a new world now. Poor health habits or preexisting conditions can mean the difference between a slight fever and cough with the coronavirus—or a ventilator and an ICU room.

So clear your schedule for one hour this week, grab a pen and paper, and keep your cell phone nearby. Here's how to do a physical self-assessment in pandemic times:

1. **Ask yourself how you're feeling.** Whenever I see patients, the first thing I always ask is how they are feeling. It sounds simple, but the answer to this question is super informative. If you can honestly say you feel great, that's wonderful. But if you feel at all achy, tired, burned out, or bummed out—or have been dealing with dizziness, pain, muscle weakness, gastrointestinal problems, or a number of other ailments—that's a sign that something might be wrong. Use your pen and paper to write down exactly how you feel, physically and mentally. Be as honest, accurate, and thorough as you can.

2. **Take a hard look at your daily habits.** If you were a new patient of mine, I would try to get as much information as I could about your daily habits before I pulled out a blood pressure cuff or did a physical exam. How active are you on a regular basis? How many hours do you sleep on average? How much alcohol do you drink? Do you smoke or vape? Do you eat a lot of sugar, takeout meals, and/or mostly processed food? Or is your diet made up primarily of whole foods, with plenty of protein, fat, and green vegetables? Are you super stressed all the time or do you have a handle (mostly) on your mental health? Think about other habits you may have that could be affecting your physical or mental health.

   Now grab your pen and paper and make two columns—one for your healthy habits and the other for the not-so-healthy ones—and write each of your daily habits in one column or the other. Don't judge yourself—we all have issues (me included), but if we don't identify them, we can't address them. If you can't decide whether a habit is good or bad, create a third column with a question mark so you have it on hand.

3. **List any known health conditions and medications.** Are you overweight or obese? Do you know if you have high blood pressure or high cholesterol? Were you diagnosed with hypothyroidism years ago and haven't been tested since? Write it all down. Be sure to include any mental-health issues you may have been diagnosed with or believe you might have.

   Next, open up your medicine cabinet and write down any medications you take, with dose information and prescribing doctor. Nearly two-thirds of all Americans take at least one prescription drug,[12] but many don't know the drug's name, the dosage, or the reason they take it in the first place. Many patients also don't take their medication properly. Now is the time to find out what you're on, why you're on it, if you're taking the therapy properly, and whether you still need to be using the drug.

4. **Find out your medical family tree.** Pick up your cell and call Mom, Dad, Granny, Sis, Aunt Helen, Great-Uncle Jack, or anyone else who may be able to help you ascertain the health conditions that run in your family. Don't stop at the obvious ailments like cancer and heart disease. But if there is cancer, find out what kind of cancer, if and at what age your relative contracted the condition, his or her risk factors, how it was treated, and any other illnesses—physical and mental—that might have a congenital link.

5. **Review your past health experiences.** Have you had mostly positive or negative experiences with healthcare providers? Have you usually left a doctor's office feeling good about your visit? Or have you felt frustrated, overwhelmed, fearful, or distrustful?

   This exercise may seem random, but it's essential in pandemic times. Since past history informs future predictions, if you've had mostly negative medical experiences, you may be tempted to avoid the doctor altogether or not heed a physician's advice if and when you go. Recognizing you may have mental resistance when it comes to healthcare can help you overcome your limitations if and when you need to seek out or maintain medical treatment.

If you discover you have had mostly negative medical experiences, I'd suggest revisiting my earlier advice: It's all about attitude and the realization that things are different now. Unfortunately, now is not the time to put off a trip to the doctor because you're fearful or frustrated, or have had poor experiences in the past. If you don't like your primary-care doctor or whomever you've seen in the past, I would encourage you to find a new physician.

6. **Add up your coronavirus risk factors.** If you're older than sixty-five, male, and a person of color, your risk factors and the consequential precautions or actions you may need to take to survive and thrive in our new normal are different from those of a thirty-year-old white woman who is at her ideal/normal body weight. Make a list and include any preexisting conditions you know you have, including diabetes; high blood pressure; cancer, heart, lung, or kidney disease; COPD; sickle cell; or immunosuppressant conditions like HIV.

Vaping and Viruses

We know that a history of smoking traditional cigarettes can double the risk of severe illness from COVID-19.[13] But what about e-cigarettes, often (and erroneously) viewed as safer than smoking tobacco cigarettes?

In the weeks before COVID-19 hit the United States, vaping was on the national news 24/7. Every day, there was a different headline on e-cigarettes: an uptick in vaping-related deaths and lung injuries; the CDC's investigation into e-cigarettes; the national ban of some flavored vapes, which went into effect February 2020.

While these headlines may have fallen off the news cycle, none of these concerns about e-cigarettes has gone away. Today, vapers have something new to worry about: Research out of Stanford University shows that teens and young adults who vape are five times more likely to be diagnosed with COVID-19.[14] Why? Researchers say vaping damages the lungs, while those who use e-cigarettes are more likely to touch their face and share devices.

Another reason to drop the pen: In April 2020, at the initial height of the pandemic, the CDC found that vaping-related lung injuries were still occurring at an alarming rate, but were manifesting very similarly to COVID-19 infections, with symptoms like shortness of breath, fever, and chills.[15]

THE PANDEMIC PHYSICAL: WHAT YOU NEED TO KNOW

There is no national recommendation being made by a major health organization that everyone needs to get a physical now. And the term *pandemic physical* is my own. But the concept conveys my point: I think nearly everyone should strongly consider getting a comprehensive medical checkup now, especially if you haven't been to the doctor in the past year. An annual checkup with a qualified healthcare practitioner, regardless of what you want to call it, is the best way to make sure your health is in order and you have no sneaky chronic conditions that could increase your risk of serious illness or death.

Take this consideration seriously: No matter who you are or how you feel, preexisting conditions are far more common than you think. Sixty percent of all Americans have at least one chronic health condition.[16] Two-thirds of all Americans are overweight or obese. One in three American adults has prediabetes. Nearly half of all adults have high blood pressure. And the list goes on.

One of the biggest benefits of a pandemic physical is that it can help unearth a risky chronic condition that you didn't know you have. I see prediabetes, high cholesterol, and mental illness in my patients all the time—every single week. And the overwhelming majority of them tell me they had no clue or never even fathomed that they had the condition.

None of this is meant to frighten you, but to encourage you to make an appointment with your doctor or healthcare provider. Remember, this is a judgment-free zone: If you haven't been to the doctor in years, don't beat yourself up or be intimidated to "find out the truth." I'm a doctor and even I fall short sometimes on my annual mammogram or skin-cancer screening. But now is the time to act and correct the problem. Here's how to get a comprehensive pandemic physical:

1. **Make the appointment already.** The best place to start is with your primary-care doctor, but if you don't have one, an OB-GYN, internist, family medicine doc, nurse practitioner, or physician's assistant can also perform a comprehensive checkup. Don't be afraid to find a new doctor if you're not comfortable with your current practitioner. Think of it this way: If you didn't like a certain food as a kid, would you give

up on all food altogether? No, you'd just avoid that specific food and find ones you like better. It's the same with physicians and just as important for your overall well-being.

2. **Discuss your self-assessment.** Don't assume every doctor will ask you every question that he or she should. Some doctors are better than others, while many simply don't have the time or bandwidth to be as thorough as they should be, unfortunately. That's why it's up to you to bring up important topics like your family history, medication regimen, "not so healthy" habits, symptoms that might indicate a preexisting condition, and other concerns that you discovered during your self-assessment. Be sure to include any mental-health concerns, too—these are just as critical to your overall health as any physical issues.

3. **Look for problems, not praise.** The point of having a pandemic physical isn't to get a glowing review from your doctor, but to find possible problems so you can do something to fix them. This was the attitude I had when I went to parent-teacher conferences when my children were young. Don't just tell me that my kid is amazing—tell me what they need to work on so we can all benefit and grow.

4. **Ask your doc about your weight.** Most physicians don't discuss body weight with patients, despite the fact that this measurement is one of the biggest risk factors for most diseases—and the single biggest chronic risk factor for COVID-19. Don't be afraid to ask your doctor if he or she thinks your weight, BMI, or body-fat composition (if your physician can take this measurement) is unhealthy. If so, ask if he or she would recommend medication or surgery.

5. **Have your blood pressure checked in *both* arms.** This is a pet peeve of mine. Most practitioners check blood pressure in only one arm, which doesn't give an accurate snapshot

of a patient's hypertension risk. Ask your practitioner to check both arms, with an appropriate size blood pressure cuff, which is what's recommended by the American Heart Association.

6. **Get poked.** Almost every annual physical, especially one performed in pandemic times, should include bloodwork to rule out the possibility of diabetes, infection, and other disorders or diseases. You don't need to be fasting or have twenty different panels performed. Just be sure that your bloodwork includes a:

   • Hemoglobin A1C test, which shows how much glucose your red blood cells have been exposed to in the last thirty days
   • Basic metabolic panel, which checks for kidney and liver function
   • Complete blood count, or CBC, which helps assess your overall health and inflammation levels
   • Lipid panel, to check both bad and good cholesterol (LDL and HDL, respectively) and your triglycerides. You don't need to be fasting to check LDL/HDL, but your triglycerides could be affected if you are not fasting.

7. **Follow up.** If you can't view the results of your bloodwork online, ask for a copy so you can review and share with other healthcare providers if necessary. Ideally, your doctor should call you to discuss the results, especially if they include any alarming numbers (often flagged in red on your results, helping patients to detect possible problems). If your doctor doesn't call, feel empowered to call his or her office. After all, it's your time, your money, and most important, your life.

If you learn you have a chronic condition, especially one like diabetes that will make you more vulnerable to COVID-19:

» **Don't freak out.** Chronic conditions are common. What matters most is that you found the problem and are now going to do something to address it.

» **Schedule a follow-up appointment with your doctor or a specialist.** Never try to treat yourself with Google Search. Medical misinformation is as prolific online as computer cookies. It's important to discuss your condition with a trained healthcare provider who can help you make informed decisions about how to best treat the ailment.

» **Focus on food and fitness.** You may not get a prescription to eat less sugar and move more, but diet and exercise are just as important as prescription drugs, if not more so, in reducing the symptoms and presence of most chronic diseases. A majority of chronic conditions, including type 2 diabetes and high blood pressure, are reversible through food and fitness.

» **Prioritize adding, not subtracting.** Many chronic conditions can be addressed by changing your diet. If you're diagnosed with high blood pressure, for example, your doc will likely ask you to reduce your intake of high-sodium foods. But I like to remind my patients with hypertension that they can also eat more high-potassium foods (like broccoli, watermelon, and avocados). Focusing on what you can eat, not what you *can't* eat, can help you better adhere to a new nutritional plan.

» **Cut down on alcohol and stress.** There's no chronic condition that benefits from too much booze or stress, period. Both increase inflammation and can cause a disease to develop in the first place. While alcohol intake has become more prodigious during the pandemic, all that beer, wine, and liquor is hurting, not helping, your ability to get through tough times, no matter what you may think. Similarly, while stress levels can redline during a pandemic, you can still learn how to keep your anxiety under control. For more on how to deal with alcohol and stress, read chapter 2: Mind.

In the new normal, what you do with your body matters more than ever before. You have an amazing opportunity right now to use COVID-19 as your wake-up call to get as physically healthy as possible, not only for this pandemic but also for the next one down the road. I know it's not easy working on your health, especially if you're suffering from more than one chronic condition. But whether our world is facing another outbreak, you get diagnosed with another condition later in life, you feel anxious, stressed, or depressed, or you simply want to be able to do all the things you love with the people you love for the longest amount of time, improving your body is one of the best ways to become more resilient.

CHAPTER 2

Mind

At the beginning of the pandemic, when we still believed the coronavirus was largely contained to Wuhan, China, Dr. Anthony Fauci stated that the risk to the American public was low. In the national and local media, we repeated that belief.

And it was—at the time. Many health experts, myself included, thought it was inconceivable that what was happening in China would ever happen here. We erroneously believed that the United States was better prepared, at least medically, and that while the virus would certainly come to the States, it wouldn't impact America as severely as it had Wuhan.

We were wrong, obviously. As the virus began to spread swiftly throughout Europe and made landfall in the United States, my perception changed, practically overnight. I realized that the United States was in no better shape than China to handle COVID-19, and may have been even more poorly equipped for a global health threat. The situation started to spiral quickly, as I began appearing on air up to fourteen hours a day. After I saw a picture of empty store shelves in Italy with the headline "Coming to New York City

Soon," I went on Amazon to order a month's supply of sardines, crackers, toilet paper, and other essentials.

At the end of February, news broke that the first American had died from the virus. I was called on a weekend and told to urgently phone into the studio for a special report on ABC News. I told viewers that the United States' strategy would likely have to shift immediately from one of containment to mitigation. It was like getting a tsunami warning, and while we all wanted to believe the wave would never come, we were now seeing this massive upsurge in the ocean on the horizon—and it was only getting bigger and bigger and closer and closer.

By March, I was reporting around the clock, seven days a week, listening and commenting in real time to every White House Task Force briefing and reading every study, no matter how preliminary, that was published on the virus. The advice seemed to change hour by hour, and the situation was advancing in rapid succession. At first, companies began to close and people started working from home, then New York City shut down, and my two kids came home from college to live with me—not by choice, but because their universities had suddenly shuttered.

My news reports began to take a sobering turn. It was now clear that the United States didn't have enough masks to protect healthcare workers and that there were also not enough ventilators to protect the lives of all the Americans who might get critically ill. I reported on air as refrigerated trucks started rolling ominously into New York and New Jersey, acting as morgues to hold the growing number of dead as hospitals and funeral homes became overwhelmed. In March, we learned that the studio had a confirmed COVID-19 case. I was notified as someone with whom this person had had prolonged, close contact. Many of us went into self-quarantine, myself included, and I started broadcasting out of my apartment.

In April, we were struck a big blow at ABC: One of our colleagues, Tony Greer, a camera operator for *Good Morning America,* had died from the virus. I was saddened and horrified. That same week, my brother, also a doctor, was diagnosed with the disease, and five more people I knew personally passed away from the virus, four of them were black.

All of a sudden, I felt like I was in the eye of a perfect storm, reporting on the horrors of the virus at work while those horrors were hitting home. I was waking up at four every morning to cover the coronavirus for hours on end without any physical, mental, or emotional change. It was like being strapped into some awful emotional roller-coaster ride from which I could never get off.

Up until this point, I had been able to keep my personal fears at bay, but now I was scared for my life. If I died from COVID-19, who would take care of my kids? I was the only parent they had. My anxiety and fears began to manifest in my dreams at night. In one dream, I was intubated in the ICU, and my boyfriend, who's an infectious disease doctor in Boston, rushed to New York to be by my side. When he finally got to my bed, he tried to slip an engagement ring on my senseless finger, but it was too late: I died from COVID-19 the moment the ring sparkled on my hand.

These dreams were just one warning sign that the pandemic had started to affect my mental health. But what could I do? I couldn't snap my fingers and make the coronavirus go away. And I couldn't—nor did I want to—stop reporting on the virus and delivering the medical insight that so many had now come to rely upon.

It was then I realized that since I couldn't change any of my external factors, I had to change something inside me. My doctor brain began to kick in, and I went back to the basics I had learned in med school.

In medicine, we always use facts, not fear, and evidence, not emotions, to guide us through difficult decisions and procedures. I rely on this outlook all the time in my own practice—because while I'm a doctor on TV, I'm not just "a doctor on TV." I also see patients in real life. And when patients are frightened, whether by unfavorable test results or a grim diagnosis, I acknowledge that feeling and then use facts to help them overcome it. I tell patients what I know and the ways in which we can help them. I don't dwell on what might or could happen—I focus instead on what I know to be happening.

It was now time to apply my own patient process to myself. I had to go back to the facts—my facts. I knew I was healthy, with no underlying medical conditions, and that my risk of dying from the disease at age fifty hovered somewhere around 1 percent. I reminded myself that 80 percent of all cases are mild and don't require hospitalization. For the next several days, I repeated these numbers over and over to myself.

Less than one week later, my fear and anxiety had ebbed almost completely, and my COVID-19 nightmares had nearly subsided. It was a dramatic shift—and it saved me.

Today, despite all we've been through as a country and that I've been through personally as a doctor, mother, and daughter of two eighty-year-old parents, my fear and anxiety have never returned to that super-high level. I've adapted the best I can, mentally and emotionally, to our new normal. All this is not to say that I'm in denial or can somehow overlook the real problems the pandemic has produced, including widespread unemployment, racial inequity, financial struggle, and a staggering death toll. I couldn't ever overlook those facts. And those facts do bother me profoundly, every day. But I have learned to apply the advice that my mother, a retired nurse, has reiterated for years: *You can't control what happens. But you can control what you do with what happens.*

Remembering my mother's aphorisms and relying on "facts over fear" are some of the ways that I've used self-talk to cope with the anxiety of our new normal. These strategies may help you, too, but there are also countless other ways to deal with the mental and emotional fallout of our new normal. Throughout the pandemic, I've discovered, learned, experienced, and recommended new ways to tackle the roller-coaster ride of anxiety, stress, depression, sadness, loneliness, and/or burnout that many of us now face. I've seen firsthand how my patients, friends, colleagues, and the viewers I've spoken with on air have been able to start to heal from mental hardship. I've also read the research, reported on it, and spoken extensively with leading experts about how pervasive mental-health problems are right now—what many psychiatrists now call the world's "second pandemic."

If you're thinking you don't have any mental-health hardships to contend with, I'd encourage you to reconsider. As I said in the introduction, the pandemic has been too disruptive, terrifying, and traumatic for all of us not to have some degree of post-traumatic stress disorder right now. What's more, almost everyone has experienced a loss since 2019. Your loss may be obvious—a loved one, your job, your home, or your business—or more subtle, like your freedom to travel, see friends and family with abandon, exercise in a gym, or maintain relationships with those who don't share your same risk tolerance. But we've all endured some kind of loss—and it's critical to recognize and grieve that loss. If you don't, you may never get over it, allowing the trauma of the pandemic to haunt you for months to come.

But what's just as important as healing from our past losses is learning to cope with what we've been left with today, which is life in our new normal. Depending on your situation, you may be so stressed with work, family, or financial anxieties that you haven't even had time to consider how the new normal is impacting you. Conversely, you might live alone and have all the time in the world to think about the trials and tribulations of a new normal. How you feel about our new reality might be subtle, too. Michelle Obama, for example, announced that she was now suffering from a "low-grade depression" due to the pandemic—something that many can probably relate to.

The bottom line is that it's important to be honest with yourself about how the new normal is affecting you. There are few constants in our lives right now, and that uncertainty isn't going away—when and if the coronavirus pandemic ends, we always face the possibility of another outbreak. Amid all this change, our emotions are collateral damage. Destabilizing feelings have been with us for many months now—one reason people who have never struggled with mental-health issues are now experiencing them every day. Understanding how the pandemic era is affecting you, mentally and emotionally, can help you address the anxiety and discover a new level of mental health, happiness, and resiliency.

In this chapter, I want to give you as many keys as possible to help you find the one that will unlock a new level of mental health, happiness, and resiliency for you. Using what I know as a doctor and have learned on the front lines of this pandemic from Day One, along with principles I've learned from mental-health professionals, I want to show you the ways in which you can accept what you can't control and control what you can. Wishful thinking won't return your life to the old normal. Instead, I encourage you to reframe your mindset and accept our new normal so you can face the present—and the future—with optimism and serenity.

THIS IS WHAT A SECOND PANDEMIC LOOKS LIKE

You've likely seen the statistics and read the headlines. The United States is facing a second pandemic—this time, an outbreak of mental illness—with tens of millions of Americans falling sick from psychological trauma.

The headlines began appearing only weeks after the virus emerged in the United States. In April 2020, nearly half of all Americans said the pandemic was negatively impacting their mental health.[1] Calls to federal emergency hotlines for those in emotional distress shot up by 1,000 percent.[2] Anxiety and depression became widespread, as researchers estimated half of all Americans were suffering from depressive symptoms.[3] Alcohol sales and substance abuse skyrocketed, along with reports of domestic abuse and violence. In May 2020, the World Health Organization (WHO) warned of a "massive increase in mental health issues in the coming months."[4] Doctors began to see spikes in the kind of post-traumatic stress disorder (PTSD) typically associated with war, physical violence, and natural disaster.[5]

But this was unlike war, destructive hurricanes, 9/11, or other historically traumatic events. The coronavirus pandemic had no discernible enemy. It had no safe zones or areas out of harm's way. And perhaps worst of all, it had—and has—no end in sight.

This reality, in turn, has caused what researchers have called "life-altering short-term and likely long-term effects" on our mental health.[6] *Life-altering* is a strong word for scientists to use, but it's not hyperbole. Think about that for a moment.

On an international scale, the pandemic has triggered a new level of fear unlike anything the world has ever seen before, with nearly every person on the planet fearful for his or her life or family's lives at one point or another. The way the virus has sickened and killed—both prodigiously and indiscriminately—has caused crippling uncertainty, as the realization has sunk in that no one is 100 percent safe.

For me, the universality of this anxiety hit home after many at ABC were exposed to a confirmed COVID-19 case. For the next several weeks, as we self-quarantined, I fielded questions from dozens of colleagues who were worried sick that they had the virus. And I mean really worried. Nearly everyone told me they had chest tightness, which I eventually realized wasn't due to COVID-19, but to the overwhelming anxiety we were all feeling.

As the pandemic progressed, anxiety over individual survival combined with other concerns. Millions of Americans lost their jobs, creating widespread financial panic, as schools closed, leaving families scrambling to find childcare and keeping older students from following their dreams. Many were forced to work from home, which has produced its own anxieties, and nearly everyone's daily routine has been disrupted. Almost every outlet, whether you like to travel, dine out, see a show, go to the gym, or even go outside for a walk, has been either stripped away or transformed.

Through it all, many have lost something far greater than the ability to travel or even work a job: They've lost a loved one to COVID-19.

Regardless of what any of us has faced or lost, we've all had to do it seemingly alone. We've experienced lockdown or stay-at-home orders—and it's possible that many of us will have to do it again. We've been cut off from family, friends, and colleagues. Few have been able to share joy, and almost no one has been able to share pain, with no funerals, family get-togethers, or in-person support groups.

This kind of isolation has sparked an epidemic of loneliness, which psychologists say could take years to recede.[7] Not only a mental-health crisis, it's also a physical-health crisis: Loneliness is known to increase the risk of premature death[8] and can be as detrimental to overall health as smoking up to fifteen cigarettes per day.[9]

The pandemic's toll has been felt by people of all ages, races, and socioeconomic classes. Yet the effects have been especially detrimental to those who had mental-health issues before the coronavirus crisis struck. Many have deteriorated—and will continue to deteriorate as the pandemic drags on. Rehab centers have also reported a spike in relapses in those dealing with alcohol or drug problems.[10]

Another sector of the population more prone to mental-health issues is those who have recovered from COVID-19. We now know that the virus can leave some with long-haul COVID-19 syndrome or post-intensive care syndrome (PICS), triggering anxiety, sleep problems, depression, or PTSD.[11] Even those who don't receive intensive care or hadn't had severe COVID-19 can develop these conditions.[12]

In other words, we've all been affected—some in more ways than others—and the extent of the pandemic's mental-health impact may take years to overcome.

While it may be comforting to think none of the mental-health problems prompted by the pandemic affects you, everyone has been impacted in one way or another. That's because every single one of us has lost something. Maybe you lost your job or the career that defined you. Maybe you lost your sense of community, daily routine, ability to travel, or another personal pastime. Maybe you even lost a friend, colleague, or family member to the virus. But we've all lost something.

At the very least, no matter who you are, where you live, or what you like to do, everyone has lost a sense of normalcy. And this is a real and profound loss.

Even my mother has been moved to tears multiple times because she says she doesn't recognize the world she lives in anymore—and at age eighty, her world isn't very wide right now. That's the degree to which the pandemic has changed what's normal. And while some aspects of our pre-pandemic lives have already resumed or will continue to do so, in other ways nothing will ever be the same again.

My point is: You don't have to have a clinical diagnosis of depression, anxiety, or traumatic stress disorder to be suffering now. You simply have had to live through the pandemic.

In May 2020, when everything was unraveling, I remember saying to *GMA3* co-anchor Amy Robach that what I found particularly unnerving was that everyone's emotional support network had suddenly shattered at a time when we needed that support the most. After I lost my ex-husband to suicide, for example, I went through some of the darkest days of my life. But despite the pain, what comforted me was knowing that others around me were strong. During the pandemic, we can't rely on someone else's strength because we're all going through the same thing: We're all dealing with loss.

What Grief Can Look Like

If you believe you haven't been emotionally impacted by the coronavirus crisis, you may be in denial—the first of the five stages of grief, first proposed by Elisabeth Kübler-Ross. While the once-popular model is no longer widely used among psychiatrists— we've learned that people process grief differently and some even skip stages[13]—knowing a little about each stage can help you confront and eventually overcome your emotions:

- *Denial:* Refusing to accept a loss has occurred can help some minimize the initial pain and shock.
- *Anger:* Suffering through a loss can cause some to feel angry, frustrated, irritable, and/or anxious. Some may also look to place blame for the loss.
- *Bargaining:* This can occur when some begin to negotiate with themselves or a higher power to help mitigate the pain. For example, some might bargain by vowing, "Please, God, if I don't get sick now, I'll promise to start taking care of my health immediately" or "Once this is over, I'll change X, Y, or Z."
- *Depression:* Some will feel a sense of sadness once the reality of the loss sets in.

- *Acceptance:* Eventually, most will accept the loss and realize that they will be okay.

It's also important to recognize that it may take some people months or even years for the reality of our new normal to sink in. Just as this crisis impacts everyone differently, it also has a way of landing on people's timelines that is both unpredictable and deeply personal.

LOOKING IN AND LIVING OUT

Since the beginning of the outbreak, you've likely experienced a range of emotions—perhaps even more than once. Because our emotions have changed so much and everyone experiences things differently in his or her own time, there is no one-size-fits-all advice for the mental health struggles you may be facing.

But just like the human spirit is universal, there are some universal truths in how we can address our emotions. The first group of strategies in this section are internal, meaning they can help you find the strength within to help you heal and build resilience. The second group of strategies are external, designed to help you connect with others outside yourself who can help steer you back to solid ground. I've used every single one of these strategies at different times and would encourage you to experiment to find the combination that works best for you.

Self-Talk for Pandemic Living

In our new normal, where things often feel upside down or uncertain, what you tell yourself is key to keeping your emotions in check. Self-talk requires self-honesty, though, along with the recognition that whatever you're feeling is okay. Try not to judge yourself, fight your feelings, or pretend those emotions aren't there. To heal, you need to be honest with yourself about what you are experiencing. There is no wrong answer.

Acknowledge your loss. We've all suffered loss. The first step in mourning that loss is to recognize that it happened and that any negative emotions you might feel now exist for a reason. You don't need to dwell on your loss, but don't minimize or sugarcoat it, either. Acknowledgment opens the door to acceptance.

Accede to uncertainty. I've said it on air multiple times: No one has a crystal ball. No one knows what will happen tomorrow—or two weeks or two years from tomorrow. This has always been true, but it's even more applicable in a pandemic. Neither you nor I nor even Dr. Anthony Fauci knows how this will end or what our world will look like in the future. And that's okay.

Acceding to uncertainty can help you stop searching for answers in a cloudy crystal ball. It can help you learn to enjoy the moment and look to the future with open arms. What will be, will be. The future could be wonderful, it could be challenging, or it could be both, but that's the beauty of life: When nothing is sure, everything is possible.

Choose facts over fear. This simple mantra helped me overcome my own fears and anxiety. While raw emotions like sorrow, loneliness, and anxiety may feel real, they're not based in facts—they're your responses to a situation or set of circumstances. Identifying and focusing on what you know to be true instead of letting what you think or feel might be true can help change how you respond.

For example, if you're feeling anxious because you've lost your job, reevaluate your own set of facts. Is there a way to earn a living that you're choosing not to pursue for some reason? Is there a way to use this as an opportunity to remake yourself or reenter the workforce at a higher level? Your answers are the facts. You don't have to act on them, but identifying and reminding yourself of the evidence can turn unpleasant emotions into inner peace.

Replace grief with gratitude. When we suffer a loss, no matter the scope, it leaves a hole in our hearts. We can either wallow in it or start to heal that hole by replacing our grief with gratitude. It can be difficult to be thankful in challenging times, but we can all find things to be grateful for, whether it's your health, a roof over your head, a special relationship with a friend, or even the ability to purchase and read a book.

You can also be grateful for the same thing you're grieving—in fact, doing so can help you recover from a loss more quickly. For example, you may be upset that you can't see your family in person, but you can be grateful that you have family in the first place.

Let it RAIN. This easy-to-remember acronym, created by psychologist Tara Brach, stands for Recognize, Allow, Investigate, and Nurture, which means recognize your feelings; allow them to exist; investigate why you're feeling this way; and nurture yourself with self-compassion. It's one of the most useful tools I've found that can help me slow down whenever I feel my thoughts or feelings are spinning out of control.

RAIN may sound simple, but when you recognize your feelings, allow them to exist, and try to view your pain from a different perspective, you open yourself up to a new level of awareness and the fact that you are hurting. You can then try to give yourself the compassion you need, whether it's in the form of forgiveness, reassurance, or simply self-love.

Avoid self-soothing. Sales of booze and comfort foods like cookies and chips skyrocketed soon after the pandemic hit. While indulging in either can seem like a way to avoid pain and uncertainty, consuming too much alcohol or junk food usually just intensifies our troubles after the initial buzz of booze or sugar wears off. What's more, drinking too much or eating too much sugar can harm your physical health, potentially making you more suscep-tible to COVID-19.

Establish a routine. After your whole world shatters, creating a new safe haven can help ease your anxiety and loss. You likely haven't been able to resurrect the daily routine you had before the pandemic, and that's okay. Instead, just create a new routine and stick to it.

Minimize the news. This may sound surprising coming from someone who delivers the news daily, but watching or reading media 24/7 might drag you down deeper into the depths of despair, according to mental-health professionals. Try unplugging for a few days to assess whether it buoys you up, mentally or emotion-ally. When I took on a mini staycation in July 2020, I didn't turn on my television once or check news on my phone for nine days. I felt much more relaxed, not only because I wasn't working around the clock, but also because I wasn't engaging in the emotional overload news can trigger for some people.

Find meaning in life's little things. Several months after the pandemic hit, I found myself taking real pleasure in previously pedestrian activities like cutting the grass and cooking a new meal. Since I wasn't able to accomplish things in other areas of my life, I realized that these everyday projects had taken on new meaning, especially when they offered a visceral sense of accomplishment, like seeing a freshly cut lawn or tasting a delicious new dish. Since then, I've learned to celebrate more of life's little victories.

When to Get Help

If you've suffered from clinical depression, anxiety, post-traumatic stress disorder (PTSD), or another mental-health illness in the past—or fear you might be experiencing an acute mental-health issue now—all the looking inward and living outward you can do may not be enough to help you heal. If you're struggling, I would encourage you, whether you have a history of mental illness or not, to get help from a psychiatrist, psychologist, social worker, licensed therapist, or trained mental-health professional. There is no shame in asking for help—everyone needs a little from time to time, including doctors like me. Don't know if you need help for a mental-health issue? If you're considering the possibility, there's no harm in speaking with a mental-health professional who can help you decide what you might need.

Healing Yourself with Help from Others

No one is an island unto themselves. We're all human beings, and by our nature, we require connections with others to survive. While learning to heal yourself from within is crucial, looking to others to help you heal is incredibly important, if not imperative. Everyone, and I do mean *everyone,* needs help outside themselves. Here are a few tools to help you reach out to get the help you need:

Know that you're not alone. You may not be able to rely on others for strength and support, but you can rely on them for solidarity. We've all been through the same thing, and we're all grieving. You're not alone in this, which can be a comforting realization.

Connect with friends and family. Human beings are social animals, and we crave connection with others. While it can be tempting to recoil inward when we're hurting, doing so won't help our physical, mental, or emotional health. Reach out to family, friends, colleagues, and neighbors as often as you can, even if it's just to say hi.

Connect with strangers. You've heard the saying *Practice ran-*

dom acts of kindness. While doing so can make others feel good, it can also make *you* feel good. In other words, you don't have to rely only on friends and family for social connection. Random acts of kindness can be small, like thanking restaurant and grocery store employees every time you see them, or remembering the name of the postal worker or delivery person you see every week. Also consider volunteering, whether through virtual channels or in person.

Connect with animals. While we're social creatures by nature, being with other human beings isn't the only way in which we can fulfill our innate need to connect. There's a good reason people cleaned out pet shelters during the pandemic: Animals can help satisfy our inner social animal and heal depression, anxiety, loneliness, and other forms of emotional trauma.

Staying Sane as a Parent in Pandemic Times

If you're a parent, this pandemic hasn't been easy. I know myself—I have two kids who lived with me for months during the initial outbreak. While both Alex and Chloe are college-age, they're still my babies, and our new normal has presented us as a family unit with a whole new set of emotional challenges and issues.

No matter how old your children are, you likely face a degree of anxiety over their health, along with uncertainty about how to best help them stay safe and deal with their own emotions in our new normal. In chapter 9, I'll walk you through how to address each age group—whether your child is a toddler, young kid, preteen, or teenager, or in college—and the ways you can help them stay safe and feel safe right now.

Just remember that their mental health depends partially

on you. How you navigate the new normal will help to set the tone for them. Resilience, after all, is a learned behavior. While it may be challenging to be strong for yourself, try to be strong for them—sometimes having a cause larger than ourselves is all we need to break through our own emotional barriers.

THE ORGANIZATIONAL PATH TO RESILIENCY

I met philanthropist Judith Rodin several years ago at a retreat for women in California. We were both speakers at the event, and I was enraptured by what she had to say. Judith has been the first woman president of an Ivy League institution (1994–2004), the president of the Rockefeller Foundation (2005–2017), and a thought leader for years, but it was her book *The Resilience Dividend: Being Strong in a World Where Things Go Wrong* (Public Affairs, 2014) that really grabbed me.

Rodin's book explores how organizations, cities, companies, and communities can build strength and resiliency after catastrophic events, and I've been leaning on her ideas since the pandemic began. As a doctor, I knew her platform could be beneficial to individuals, too, and I've spent hours rereading her book, thinking about her guidance, and even talking about her strategy on TV.

In the book, Rodin lays out five characteristics that can help organizations build resiliency. While some apply more specifically to cities, companies, and communities, there are two that I feel are extremely apt for the individual in the world we live in now:

>> Awareness of your circumstances, strengths, and weaknesses

>> Adaptability to fast-changing conditions[14]

The first tenet—awareness of your circumstances, strengths, and weaknesses—is the basic premise of medicine. Every clinical patient evaluation starts like this, as doctors assess patients' circumstances—how they're feeling, their vital signs, their past medical history—and their medical strengths and weaknesses based on those circumstances.

When it comes to your mental and emotional health, you can apply the same approach—again, I want to encourage you to think like a doctor. So take a look at your circumstances: Are you living alone? Did you lose your job? Do you have a network of friends with whom you can connect? Are you prone to anxiety or do you have a history of psychiatric issues? Now, assess your strengths and weaknesses: If you're living alone, you're more isolated than someone who lives with family or roommates. At the same time, if you have a close, connected network of friends, that strength can help mitigate the effects of isolation. Identifying circumstances, strengths, and weaknesses can help you play into your assets and address drawbacks before they become difficulties.

The second tenet—being able to adapt quickly—is critical in a pandemic. As we've seen with the coronavirus crisis, things can change by the hour. That means we have to be ready and willing for whatever comes our way, rolling with it rather than allowing it to break us. Can't see your friends or family in person? Don't let it paralyze you but find new ways to connect remotely. Can't work in a traditional office environment? Accept it and then try to turn your home—in whatever way you can—into a space that may be even better than your old office.

USING SELF-CARE TO SELF-HEAL

While I am always still learning, I do know a thing or two about self-care—in fact I wrote a bestselling book on the topic: *The Self-*

Care Solution: A Year of Becoming Happier, Healthier, and Fitter—One Month at a Time (HarperCollins, 2019). Even though I penned it before the pandemic hit, the advice inside has helped me considerably through the coronavirus crisis. If there was ever a time to stop, breathe, and nurture yourself, it is now.

First, let's clear up some confusion. Lots of people are baffled by what self-care actually is—and rightfully so. Like lots of buzzwords (e.g., intermittent fasting, CBD, keto), the term has been misused, overused, and inaccurately portrayed. To me, the concept means taking the time to care for your psyche like a doctor or nurse would care for a patient. That may seem like self-help, but it's not. Self-help, which was all the rage in the 1980s, implies that something inside you needs to be helped or fixed. With self-care, nothing needs to be fixed: You just need to be nurtured.

How to best nurture yourself, then? There are countless ways to practice self-care, and just like every patient is unique, every body and soul is special. In other words, you don't have to practice the same kind of self-care that your friend, colleague, or personal trainer does. Experiment to discover what best nurtures you and embrace it.

Here are three areas in which to practice care, with my top suggestions of activities to try:

1. **Nourish your body.** I believe that when your spirit is hurting, your body can help it heal. Here are some ways you can help nourish your body:
   - **Eat what you know you need.** While curling up with a pint of ice cream or bag of chips might be appealing now, it's not nourishing—and not what your body truly needs to feel good. Remember, self-care means treating your body like a doctor would a patient—and chocolate chip cookie dough ice cream is not on the prescription pad. We'll discuss the best ways to eat right for the pandemic in chapter 4 (page 79).

- **Move more.** Physical activity is one of the most effective ways to self-care, with the ability to improve your body, mood, and mind. You don't have to run a 5K or do an hour-long online aerobics class to benefit—simply taking more steps can help. For more on what you need to know about exercise in the pandemic age, see chapter 5 (page 101).
- **Hit the snooze button.** What body doesn't love a good eight hours? Give yourself the gift of delicious sleep now—because everything looks and feels better after a full night's rest. For more on how to sleep more soundly in our new normal, turn to chapter 6 (page 119).
- **Stop, stretch, and roll.** Stretching can release tension, relax your body, and help you feel more mindful. Not into stretching? Try foam-rolling, which is, in my opinion, the cheapest and easiest form of muscle massage.
- **Drink water.** This is like remembering to water household plants—it's easy to forget on a regular basis, but it can make all the colors of the world look brighter.

2. **Nourish your mind.** While many people think of self-care as something you do, what you think and how you feel are just as important—and can be just as restorative. Here are some ways to nourish your mind:
   - **Engage in a hobby that makes you happy.** It sounds simple, but few actually take the time to pursue hobbies when they're hurt, sad, lonely, or anxious. Allow yourself the time and energy to do what you enjoy, whether it's painting, playing an instrument, or gardening.
   - **Challenge your mind.** Nothing may be better than a good cognitive game to help distract your mind and enable your brain to see your problems in a new light.

Try learning a new language, doing a crossword or
jigsaw puzzle, or reading a good book.

- **Take a minute (or ten) to meditate.** Meditation is one
  of the most effective ways to help treat depression and
  anxiety, with studies showing the practice works as
  well as antidepressants for some mood disorders. Look
  online for tips on how to meditate and make it part of
  your new daily routine.
- **Write it all down.** Journaling is like venting for the soul,
  except you don't need anyone around to do it. Write
  down anything you want: what bothers you, what
  you're grateful for, what you've been through, what
  you hope to accomplish. Your journal is your space, and
  there's no write (ha!) or wrong way to use it.
- **Stop with the screens already.** With so many of us
  working from home, it's easy to stay glued to our
  screens 24/7. But easy doesn't mean healthy. Taking
  a tech break whenever possible can help refresh your
  mind and mood.
- **Laugh, giggle, chuckle, or guffaw.** You've probably
  heard it before: Laughter is the best medicine. There's
  medical research to support this maxim, with studies
  showing a good guffaw can help cut stress, boost
  happiness, and even improve the body's immune
  system. I think everyone should laugh every day,
  whether it's by watching a favorite comedy show or
  being silly with friends or family. One of the biggest
  lessons I learned during my year of self-care in *The Self-
  Care Solution* was how to laugh at myself—and that's
  truly a gift that keeps on giving!

3. **Nourish together.** We often think of self-care as a solitary
   activity, but there's no reason why you have to go it alone all

the time. As long as you're emphasizing the "self" in self-care and not doing what someone else wants or thinks you should do, there's no harm in engaging in activities with others. In fact, there may be some serious benefits to communal self-care, including creating feelings of community and connectedness—two things we all need right now. Here are some ways to practice communal self-care:

- **Take an online or outdoor yoga class.** Or any type of group fitness. This way, you nourish your body and mind while connecting with others.
- **Watch a movie, stream a ballet or Broadway show, or visit a virtual museum together.** There's nothing like savoring great art with someone else. Share the experience in whatever way you can and take the time to discuss your experience together afterward.
- **Connect with your inner circle.** Get your family or live-in household together for a special night of cooking, playing board games, watching (or re-watching) a big sports match, or otherwise doing a group activity you wouldn't normally do on just any night.

Throughout this chapter, I've given you a number of strategies that can help you find greater mental health, happiness, and resiliency in our new normal. You may need to experiment to find the exact combination that helps you, but I have full faith you can do it. Despite all the losses we've suffered, the human spirit can prevail, especially if you believe it will. Throughout history, we've survived extraordinary hardships before—the Holocaust, 9/11, two world wars—and we've always come out on the other side with a sense of fortitude and optimism. We will do so again. You will do so again.

On a personal level, you may have already lived through times of extreme emotional adversity. In every instance, you weathered the storm—after all, you are here reading this book right now. Remember this and believe that you can weather the storm again, even if you have to walk through a lot of rain to get to the rainbow on the other side.

CHAPTER 3

Healthcare

In early April 2020, the U.S. surgeon general went on national television and told the American people that the coming week would be one of the hardest and saddest in the country's history— "our Pearl Harbor moment, our 9/11 moment."[1] At the time, New York City felt and looked like a war zone, the United States' infection curve rate had shot up over the preceding month. The surgeon general was now worried that the fallout moment had come for the country's death count to catch up.

That same week, I was home with my children, Alex and Chloe, getting ready for bed when I suddenly started to itch. Moments later, while brushing my teeth, I felt incredibly dizzy. I wasn't overly concerned, at least not at first: I'm allergic to a few ingredients found in some foods and skincare products, and I figured it was something I had eaten or used on my face. I took a Benadryl and tried not to think about it.

Fifteen minutes later, I was so light-headed that I had to lie down. I crawled into bed and called my boyfriend, who is also a doctor. Before I could tell him, he asked me what was wrong, saying I didn't sound right. I checked my Apple Watch: My pulse was in the 130s. I was now tachycardic—medical speak for having an abnormally high heart rate. Often, when our heart rate is high, it's to compensate for a very low blood pressure, right before loss of consciousness occurs.

Suddenly, my heart rate dropped below 70. My boyfriend told me to call 911.

I yelled for Alex and Chloe to come into my bedroom and asked them to call an ambulance. For the first time in my life, I was having someone else do for me what I had recommended a dozen times before. Instead of being the one to respond and help, I was now the one who needed help, and it was frightening.

Moments later, the paramedics were in my apartment. They checked my heart rate, oxygen, and blood pressure, both while I was standing up and lying down. After I learned my vitals had returned to normal, I told them I was a doctor. They asked if I wanted to go to the emergency room.

My answer? "Are you kidding? Absolutely not. I'm fine."

Here I was, possibly having a medical emergency at the height of the pandemic, and I was unwilling to go to the ER. In retrospect, I probably had had an anxiety attack or weird reaction to expired Benadryl—I'll never know for sure. Fortunately, it turned out to be nothing serious. But I was willing to take the chance that whatever I had was better than going to the ER in the middle of a pandemic.

As a doctor, I was able to make that decision—and it turned out to be the right decision. But if you're not a doctor, avoiding the ER in the exact same situation would *not* have been the right decision: If you're about to lose consciousness and it's bad enough to ask someone else to call 911, it's probably bad enough to go to the hospital.

Does this mean that you should go to the ER every time you feel unwell? Absolutely not. But it shows us how complicated decisions have become, even for doctors, about when, where, and why we seek medical attention.

In short, the coronavirus has changed healthcare and how we all think about preventative medicine, along with why and how often we go to the emergency room and the doctor's office. While some of these changes are great—the rise of telemedicine, for example, can benefit a lot of people, as I'll explain later in this chapter—other common developments we're seeing like avoiding doctor appointments and emergency room visits when necessary and not keeping children up-to-date on vaccines can be detrimental, if not life-threatening.

These choices aren't necessarily born out of negligence or ignorance, but what is now the new normal for us all: risk. In pandemic times, we have to assess risk on a regular basis and determine whether it's safe to do certain activities, which includes going to the doctor and the ER. These decisions aren't easy to make, but you don't have to be a doctor to learn how to assess risk about your own healthcare—you just need to learn how to think like one.

In this chapter, I'll tell you what I know and have learned about when to go to the emergency room in a pandemic—and when an urgent-care clinic or family physician may be the better choice. I'll also share with you my experience with telemedicine and what you need to know about using the virtual service that's replaced a lot of traditional care. I'll also tell you which medical supplies I think everyone should have at home during a pandemic.

Moreover, I'll explain why learning more about how to manage your health and in what ways can help empower you, even in the seeming chaos of a pandemic. The goal of this chapter is not to become your own physician or healthcare provider—even doctors have doctors! But I want to help you make more deliberate decisions and actions for your health and to learn how to be in the driver's seat.

THE PROBLEM WITH THE ER IS NOT THE ER

The stories started making headlines in the first few weeks of the pandemic: An otherwise healthy woman in New York City who didn't go the emergency room because she was worried about the coronavirus—the next day she had a stroke.[2]

Or a Washington state woman in her mid-fifties who waited a week to go to the hospital for the worst headache of her life due to fears over the virus—her headache turned out to be a cerebral hemorrhage (aka brain bleed) that doctors couldn't treat.[3]

Or the thirty-eight-year-old Pennsylvania man who delayed going to the hospital for chest pains because of COVID-19 concerns—he suffered a fatal heart attack in his home.[4]

These are terrible and tragic stories that represent the extreme, not the norm. But they do help illustrate a pervasive trend that experts say may take years to reverse: People are scared to go the hospital. And that's not a good thing.

According to a CDC report, emergency room visits fell by 42 percent in the weeks after the onset of the outbreak.[5] Around the same time, a study published in *The Journal of the American Medical Association* showed a big jump in the number of deaths due to diabetes, heart disease, Alzheimer's disease, and other common causes of hospital visits in states with the most COVID-19 fatalities.[6] The spike was not insignificant either, with New York City seeing a 398 percent jump in heart disease deaths and a 356 percent jump in diabetes deaths compared to years past.[7] Researchers attributed the uptick to the fact that people were afraid to go to the hospital due to the coronavirus outbreak.

Fears over COVID-19 contagion and the ER are understandable—I had them, too. But they're fears, not facts. So let's look at the facts.

Fact #1: Medical Emergencies Don't Stop Because There's a Pandemic

While everything else might come grinding to a halt when there's a viral outbreak, medical emergencies don't go on vacation just because there's a new pathogen working overtime. Appendicitis still happens during an outbreak, as do heart attacks, strokes, car accidents, and all the other reasons why people can end up in the ER. Don't get tunnel vision and think that the only threat to your health is COVID-19 (or the latest high-impact pathogen): Every ailment that was a risk before the pandemic is still a risk now—and to the same degree.

Fact #2: The Hospital Is Likely the Safest Place We Have When It Comes to COVID-19

The major breeding grounds for coronavirus that we've seen so far are cruise ships, prisons, nursing homes, and households. I want you to notice that nowhere on that list are hospitals or emergency rooms, despite the fact that we know COVID-19 exists in both places in a higher concentration than is likely in other places. That's important to remember because it's a fact, not a perception or an opinion.

Fact #3: This Isn't Your Local Emergency Room's First Rodeo

Hospitals have been dealing with patients with highly communicable diseases for years. They are well schooled in infection control practices and have entire in-house teams dedicated to rapid response measures. Hospitals are also equipped with personal protective gear, negative pressure rooms to prevent airborne transmission, and other tools and technology to help reduce the risk of other patients getting sick. In other words, hospitals can practically do COVID-19 control in their sleep.

Fact #4: The Measles Is More Contagious Than COVID-19, But No One Freaked Out About Going to the Hospital During the 2019 Outbreak

Measles is the most contagious and transmissible respiratory infection in the world, much more so than COVID-19. If you walked into a room where a person with measles had coughed hours earlier and you weren't vaccinated, there's a 90 percent chance you'd come down with the potentially deadly disease. In 2019, there was a major outbreak of measles in the United States, centered around the greater New York City metro area. But you didn't hear about people avoiding hospitals en masse, even though many measles cases were treated in area wards.

Fact #5: If Hospitals Can Handle Ebola, They Can Deal with COVID-19

Remember when the first Ebola case came to the United States in 2014? Americans erupted in fear after a man was hospitalized in Dallas, Texas, with the disease. The virus, which includes symptoms like fever, diarrhea, vomiting, and bleeding, is fatal in approximately half of all patients who become infected. After the Dallas case came out in the news, Ebola was the leading headline of every major media outlet for weeks. America's fear became so severe that then-president Barak Obama urged the public not to "give in to hysteria,"[8] in part because the hysteria was largely unfounded. With four designated Ebola treatment centers across the country at the time, the United States was trained, drilled, rehearsed, and ready to contain the infection. (By 2020, the United States had more than thirty designated treatment centers.) That's one reason we saw only eleven confirmed cases in the States of the highly contagious disease during the 2014–2016 outbreak.

Fact #6: Hospitals Aren't Waiting for the Missing Link in COVID-19 Care

Yes, the coronavirus is a new disease, and yes, we're continually learning more about the virus every day. But that doesn't mean doctors are sitting around the ER waiting for a missing piece of information in order to limit exposure to anyone who dares step inside a hospital. Infection control and patient care in the United States is based on the most up-to-date, evidence-based science—it's not based on hypotheses or expectations of a more comprehensive protocol to come. You should feel comfortable and confident that you are getting the best available care anytime you go to the hospital, even when we are dealing with a new virus.

WHEN TO GO TO THE EMERGENCY ROOM

While emergency rooms are safe places and experienced in containing infectious illnesses, no hospital is 100 percent safe for 100 percent of patients 100 percent of the time. In other words, the spread of COVID-19 can, will, and has occurred within hospital walls. Hospitals attract sick people, after all, and while doctors and nurses are trained to deal with illness, it's not always possible to ensure that every single patient or staff member knows or follows the rules all the time.

That's why it's not necessarily surprising that one study found that as many as one in five coronavirus patients in the United

Kingdom caught the virus while being treated for other illnesses at area hospitals.[9] In other words, while your risk of COVID-19 exposure at a hospital is low, it's not zero.

You also have a minimal chance of catching a host of other communicable illnesses at a hospital—which has always been true, long before the first coronavirus case was ever recorded. While the world may be COVID-centric now, hospitals see patients all the time with highly contagious illnesses like influenza, norovirus, and tuberculosis. What's more, unlike COVID-19, many patients with these types of infectious illnesses don't always know or take steps to help prevent others from also becoming infected until after they're diagnosed.

There's another persistent reason not to run to the ER every time you have a fever, feel pain, or suffer a stomachache. The ER is for emergencies—hence the name, *emergency* room. Going to the hospital for non-urgent issues takes away resources from those who need them, like all the people who have heart attacks, strokes, serious accidents, and other life- or limb-threatening events. Unnecessary hospital visits also waste money, costing up to $8.3 billion in preventable expenses every year.[10]

While some may think it's obvious the ER is for emergencies only, not everyone shares or can share this perception: Up to 30 percent of all emergency room visits are for non-critical issues that could easily be treated by an urgent-care clinic or primary-care doctor.[11] Unfortunately, however, many Americans don't have a regular healthcare provider or can't afford health insurance, relying on the ER for basic medical care. Either way, it's important that those with healthcare resources not add to the strain, especially during a pandemic when so many hospitals are already overburdened.

These are just some of the reasons to think twice about taking a trip to the ER during a pandemic. At the same time, there are plenty of reasons to rush to the hospital and prevent yourself or a loved one from joining the recent string of tragic stories about people who didn't go to the ER out of fear of catching the coronavirus. But how on earth do you make that decision? Or when do the benefits of going to the ER outweigh the possible risks, including exposure to COVID-19?

Before we get to these answers, I want to clear something up: I'm not suggesting that anyone try to manage his or her own healthcare in lieu of speaking with a doctor or healthcare professional. We don't live on the moon, after all, which means most of us have access to a clinic or a healthcare provider whom we can call or see at all hours, even at night and over the weekend (because, P.S., almost all doctors have an after-hours service).

That said, when there's a pandemic going on in the world, it pays to be able to think like a doctor and weigh the pros versus the cons of going to a crowded, potentially overburdened emergency room where you might be exposed to COVID-19 or a number of other communicable diseases.

With that understanding, here are some things to consider if and when you or a loved one is thinking about taking a trip to the hospital:

• **Call 911 for life- or limb-threatening emergencies.** If you're having chest pain, trouble breathing, standing, eating, drinking, or speaking, you've been in a serious accident, or you have acute pain that is getting worse by the hour, go to the ER immediately. These are all symptoms that could indicate a life- or limb-threatening emergency.

• **Ask yourself the unthinkable.** Another way to think about whether you need emergency care is to ask yourself whether the symptoms you're experiencing could potentially kill you. For example, a sprained ankle or sore throat isn't likely to be fatal without an immediate emergency room visit. However, chest pain or trouble breathing could be the sign of a life-threatening condition and likely merits immediate attention.

- **Make the decision with your pre-pandemic brain.** I've said it multiple times on air: If you would have gone to the ER for the same symptoms in pre-pandemic times, go now. Plain and simple.
- **Think for better or for worse.** In general—with an extra emphasis on *in general*—really serious conditions don't get better on their own. In fact, most get worse. If you're deteriorating by the hour, call 911. But if your symptoms are getting better and aren't life-threatening, consider calling your healthcare provider or going to an urgent-care clinic instead.
- **Weigh your risk factors.** Every patient is different, which is why it's difficult to make blanket generalizations about non-specific symptoms to a general population. But no one knows your body like you do, along with your own unique risk factors and individual medical history (or at least, you should know these things—see page 26 on how to conduct a pandemic self-assessment), which are all things to consider when weighing whether to go to the emergency room.

For example, if you're a man in your fifties with a history of high blood pressure and you start having chest pain, now is not the time to roll the dice on whether to go to the ER. However, if you're a healthy twenty-year-old woman with mild chest pain and zero history of heart problems, it's much less likely that you're having a traumatic event. However, if a twenty-year-old woman with arrythmia starts feeling the same mild chest pain, the game changes.

- **Focus on identifying the ducks.** There's a saying in medicine that I like to use often on air and in my medical practice: *If it looks like a duck, swims like a duck, and quacks like a duck, it's probably a duck*. In other words, if you're having similar symptoms to a condition that a doctor diagnosed you with before or have all the classic symptoms of a common ailment, it's likely that's what you have now.

For example, if you're prone to migraines and develop a headache, except maybe this one lasts a little longer, it's probable that you're having another migraine—it's not likely, however, that you have an aneurysm or brain tumor. While it can be easy to spiral into imagining worst-case scenarios, especially with the help of Google Search, I always recommend checking yourself with the simple duck test.

When the Worst Headache of Your Life May Actually Be

When patients say they are having the worst headache of their life, we doctors take that complaint very seriously. "Worst headache of life," or WHOL, is actually a medical term we use. If you find yourself using this phrase to describe your symptoms, call 911. While it's rare, the pain could indicate a cerebral hemorrhage or ruptured aneurysm.

• **Don't let zebras in through the door.** If identifying ducks isn't your thing, here's another saying I used on *The View* in the winter of 2020 about the likelihood of having the flu versus COVID-19 just because you have fever and cough: *When you hear hooves outside your door, think horses, not zebras.* In medical speak, "zebras" are rare conditions that affect a small percent of the population—think brain tumors and super rare diseases. The likelihood that you're suffering from a zebra is really low. If your symptoms aren't severe and the only reason you're considering a trip to the ER is to rule out the possibility of a zebra, I'd call your healthcare provider. Remember, common things occur commonly, and an increased risk of a rare event is still a rare event.

• **Just because you *can* do something in medicine doesn't**

mean you *should* do something. Just because you can go to the emergency room doesn't mean you should go to the ER. Sometimes, reframing your outlook is all you need to help guide you to the best decision for your health.

• **Remember that life is one big risk.** Every time you leave your house or someone you live with leaves the house, you're risking possible exposure to COVID-19, along with dozens of other pathogens. That doesn't mean that you can or should live your life in a sterilized plastic bubble. If there's ever a reason to risk potential pathogen exposure, it's to go to the ER and potentially save yourself from something possibly far worse than the coronavirus.

• **Don't be afraid to call your doc.** Every doctor's office or clinic has an answering service or a way to reach the physician or provider after hours or over the weekend. If you're unsure about the risk-benefit ratio of going to the ER for a non-life-threatening condition, call your doctor. Don't worry: You're not disturbing him or her. As a doctor, I'd much rather hear from a patient about a potential problem, no matter how minor, than receive a call from the hospital that my patient suffered a major traumatic health event because they were too intimidated to contact me.

• **Your health is in your hands.** No matter where you go, whether the ER, an urgent-care clinic, or a primary-care office, wash your hands thoroughly and keep your distance from other patients—two things we should do even when we're not facing a pandemic. I also suggest that you wear a mask if recommended or if you simply feel more comfortable with personal protective equipment. Finally, always ask for your medical records and copies of any test results when you leave so that you have them on hand and readily accessible if you need follow-up care from a different provider.

The Truth About Urgent Care

How to know when to go to an urgent-care clinic instead of the ER? Urgent-care clinics fill an important need in the United States, serving as an intermediary step between your nine-to-five doctor's office or clinic and the local hospital's emergency department. Urgent-care clinics are perfect for diagnosing non-life-threatening conditions like the flu, strep throat, and other illnesses for which you may not want to wait until Monday morning—or simply the next morning—for a diagnosis.

The reasons to go to an urgent-care clinic over the ER for these types of ailments are multifactorial. First, the risk of exposure to communicable diseases like COVID-19 is often lower in urgent-care facilities, where there are fewer sick patients overall and those who are there tend to spend less time at the clinic than they do in hospitals. Second, urgent-care clinics usually save patients time and money over a trip to the ER, which can cost you hours in wait time and thousands of dollars in deductibles or co-pays, even if you have health insurance. Finally, when you choose to go to an urgent-care clinic for ailments that aren't medical emergencies, you reduce the strain on local hospitals, allowing them to use their resources for critical care to those in your community who need it the most.

THE PROS AND CONS OF TELEMEDICINE

In March, after New Jersey issued stay-at-home orders and canceled all elective surgeries, I shut down my medical practice in Englewood and started relying on telemedicine to see patients virtually. While I had used telemedicine before, this was the first time I'd used it extensively and almost exclusively, like most doctors had to do at the beginning of the COVID-19 outbreak.

Telemedicine, which uses technology like live video streaming to diagnose and treat patients, was not particularly widespread before COVID-19 shut down nearly every family physician's office nationwide. In fact, according to a recent survey by McKinsey & Company, only 11 percent of Americans had used telehealth in 2019—fast-forward to April 2020, and 46 percent had tried telehealth in just the first two months of the pandemic.[12] Additionally, 76 percent of all patients say they are interested in trying telehealth now that the pandemic has made the service essential for continuous medical care.[13]

Despite many patients' willingness to talk to a doc online, misperceptions about telemedicine persist, mainly that the practice isn't as effective as in-person visits and that it devalues the patient-doctor relationship. While doctors obviously can't do everything by video or phone, we can diagnose, prescribe, and treat patients with a range of conditions and issues. In fact, research shows that telemedicine even helps save lives, providing immediate, around-the-clock care to patients while limiting their exposure to potentially deadly infectious diseases like COVID-19. The service can be especially beneficial to older patients, those with physical disabilities or travel limitations, and people who live in rural areas, all of whom can receive care more conveniently and rapidly through telemedicine.

Telemedicine also typically costs less than in-person visits[14] and can save some patients thousands of dollars by preventing future medical emergencies, according to studies.[15] You can also save a ton of time by scheduling a telemedicine appointment, obviating the trip to a doctor's office and any time you may spend there in a waiting room. When I was practicing almost exclusively through telemedicine, I was finally able to see patients on time because I wasn't also dealing with stacks of paperwork (it's much easier to combine digital chartwork and video calls) and a waiting room full of potentially sick people.

Punctuality wasn't the only advantage of telemedicine for me during the early pandemic. The service also allowed me to be able to physically see patients, which doctors obviously can't do over the phone (though some of my patients were actually fine with a good old-fashioned phone call). That's key, because it lets us do the subjective part of a patient visit when we look for things like whether someone appears disheveled or anxious or has any other visible clues to their overall physical and mental state.

With some patients, I also asked them to take their own vitals like temperature and heart rate, which is easier to do during a video call when I can make sure the information is being collected properly. I also used our video sessions to order remote testing if needed, review prior test results, prescribe medication, and give specific health recommendations. Live video also let me connect more intimately with my patients than I could by phone or email (although calls, texts, and emails are considered part of telehealth—a broad umbrella term that includes traditional telecommunication tools in addition to video streaming and more advanced technology).

At the same time, I'm an OB-GYN—a specialty where in-person tests and tactile physical exams are critical. These can't be administered remotely, so while there was plenty that I could still do, I was limited in my practice. During the initial outbreak, I had to ask a few patients to meet me at my office—or I sent them a culture swab through the mail—in order to run tests when I thought the matter was more urgent and telemedicine alone wasn't going to cut it.

There are other disadvantages to telemedicine, too. You can't give oxygen, run an IV, or administer other lifesaving care via telemedicine. Doctors also can't draw blood, take urine, or perform other tests that may be necessary. While some specialties like psychiatry, dermatology, and chronic disease management are better suited to telemedicine, others like obstetrics and surgery aren't. I believe there is also something irreplaceable about being in the same room as patients and being able to interact more intimately with them than a screen would ever allow.

But these drawbacks are small when you consider what telemedicine has allowed doctors to do during the pandemic: provide healthcare to millions of Americans who may have otherwise not been able to receive medical attention. This is huge—and one reason why telemedicine will only continue to expand now that the pandemic has exposed how easy, convenient, and critical the service is to our new normal.[16]

I would encourage anyone who's hesitant to use telemedicine to try it. After all, the practice, like the pandemic, isn't going away anytime soon, and as you can see, there's a host of potential advantages for the patient, including that the service reduces the risk of COVID-19 exposure while saving you time, money, and possible health complications down the road.

If you're still unenthusiastic, remember that people are often suspicious about new technology the first time they use it, then usually grateful that they gave it a shot. The first time I deposited a check online, for example, I was skeptical. *Really? I'm just going to take a picture of this check and it's going to magically end up in my bank account?* But it worked—and it's worked every time since. Today, this is how I prefer to bank, because it's easier and more convenient than going to the bank in person.

SEVEN MUST-HAVES FOR HOME HEALTH

When most of the country went into lockdown at the beginning of the COVID-19 outbreak, many Americans had no idea that they actually needed to stay at home for weeks at a time. They wiped grocery-store shelves clean of everything from refrigerated egg substitute to toilet paper to trash-can deodorizers. But amid all this panic buying, many forgot some of the most important essentials: things they needed in order to take care of their health at home, on the off chance of a major medical emergency and the very likely possibility of a minor health ailment. These essentials include not only prescription drugs but also other common medical supplies people should consider having on hand, whether we're facing a pandemic or not. Here are seven items to consider stocking up with now so that you're better prepared for whatever and whenever a health ailment might come your way:

1. **Extra Rx.** When lockdown orders went into effect early in the outbreak, millions of Americans were left scrambling to get advance refills of prescription meds in order to stay at home for weeks. Some weren't able to get the refills due to insurance problems, while others faced shortages because of increased demand and medical supply-chain issues.

   If you take a prescription drug, I recommend that you have at least two weeks' worth of extra meds at home, regardless of whether there are ever stay-at-home orders again: As we learned from the pandemic, our medical-supply chain is vulnerable, and a dozen other similar events could interfere with drug availability. Talk with your doctor about advance refills; if your insurance company refuses to pay, call and explain the reason—many insurers have and will make exceptions. Just be sure to keep extra prescription drugs in a cool, dry, secure place, away from children and teenagers.

2. **A mini pharmacy.** Prescription drugs aren't the only medical supplies that face shortages—dozens of over-the-counter (OTC) drugs like cough syrup and certain antacid formulas were also in short supply during the first few months of the

outbreak. What's more, you never know when you'll need a bottle of Pepto Bismol at two in the morning. For these reasons, I suggest stocking up on a variety of OTC drugs, even those you've never used before and think you may never need—because the time you inevitably need an OTC drug is always the time when you can't get it. Be sure to include a medication to treat pain, nausea, constipation, gas, allergic reaction (e.g., Benadryl), allergies (e.g., Claritin), itching (e.g., hydrocortisone cream), skin infection (e.g., bacitracin), acid reflux, nasal congestion, and diarrhea.

3. **Two thermometers.** Drugstores sold out of thermometers just days after the first coronavirus case was identified in the United States. This left many without the ability to measure one of the symptoms of the virus, which is also a classic sign of many other ailments, including the flu, an adverse reaction to a medication, and heatstroke, among others.

    While you're stocking up, be sure to buy not one, but two thermometers. It's underreported, but thermometers can be wildly inaccurate. For example, when my daughter, Chloe, went to get a COVID-19 screening before an ice-hockey camp, she had her temperature checked at a drive-through facility with a forehead gun. The nurse told her she had a fever of 101.9, even though she felt perfectly fine and had no symptoms of COVID-19, let alone any other illness. A second reading on a different device proved that her temperature was totally normal.

4. **A smartwatch, digital fitness tracker, wristwatch, or pulse oximeter.** One reason I like wearing my smartwatch is that it makes checking my heart rate super simple and convenient—all you have to do is look down at the device. But you don't need a smartwatch or digital fitness tracker to keep tabs on your pulse—something you may want to do during a pan-

demic, as variations in heart rate can indicate a range of health problems, even when you have other obvious symptoms. For example, a resting heart rate above 100 beats per minute or below 50 beats per minute can be a sign of a heart problem, infection, medication overdose, thyroid issue, or other ailment that may warrant medical attention.

You can also check your heart rate using a pulse oximeter, a small electronic device that slips on your finger and uses light to measure your body's blood-oxygen levels. Apple's watch also checks the oxygen saturation in your blood. Pulse oximeters have become popular since the pandemic as a way for people to measure their respiratory health at home—just be aware that most oximeters don't provide a very accurate oxygen reading.

You can also check your heart rate using an old-fashioned wristwatch: Simply find your carotid artery on the side of your neck, place your index and middle finger over the spot, and count the number of heartbeats for a full minute.

5. **Basic first-aid kit.** The joke in my household is that we have five doctors in the family plus one retired nurse, yet there are times when you can't even find a Band-Aid in my home. That's not a good idea. Cuts, falls, bug bites, and other accidents happen and can worsen without some simple first aid—which is why every office, restaurant, and public building usually has some kind of first-aid kit somewhere on the premises. Be sure your kit includes rubbing alcohol, hydrogen peroxide, gauze pads, medical tape, Band-Aids, an ice pack that can be kept in the refrigerator, sterile eye wash, scissors, tweezers, and disposable gloves, among other items.

6. **Contact list.** When there's a medical emergency at home, don't trust that you'll remember who to call—or be physically well enough to find out. Keep a medical contacts list

with your primary-care physician, local pharmacy, and other emergency contacts in your smartphone and on paper (in case your phone dies or you're physically incapable of accessing it). It also helps to have a written and digital list of the medications you're taking and their prescribed doses, along with any known drug allergies, that you or a loved one can bring to the ER or share with paramedics or other healthcare providers.

7. **Medical emergency plan.** Don't wait until the unthinkable happens to consider where you or a loved one might want to go in the event of a medical emergency. Know which hospital is the closest or where you'd prefer to receive care and include the address in your medical contact list. Keep a "go bag" in your closet that includes a change of clothes, a day or two of extra medication, and anything else you might need for a short period of time if you suddenly have to go to the hospital.

Everything you've learned in this chapter isn't designed to replace the insight, advice, and care that a doctor or other healthcare practitioner can provide. But you now have some of the strategies that we doctors use to assess risk and stay safe when we seek (or don't seek) medical attention. If you can leverage these tools and start to think like a doctor, you can take some control over your own healthcare—because, ultimately, how effective and successful your healthcare will be is up to you. And in crisis times, knowing how to manage your healthcare can not only help you stay safe, but it may even save your life, as well.

CHAPTER 4

Food

When New York City first went into lockdown, I wasn't caught off guard. We had planned for it at ABC, and the network quickly set up a studio in my apartment where I could broadcast up to thirteen hours per day. We had also planned for it as a family, and Alex, Chloe, and Chloe's boyfriend, Billy, came home to live with me after their colleges abruptly closed and stay-at-home orders were issued.

Even though I was prepared to work and stay at home, I didn't foresee the effects that the lockdown would have on other areas of my life, particularly my eating. Suddenly I was working from home, within steps of my kitchen, and living with three college kids who ate more than I've ever seen human beings consume. All this was also taking place in an apartment smaller than some people's living rooms.

For those who don't know New York City living, picture the apartment you saw on *Friends* and cut it into quarters. In most Manhattan apartments, you can walk from the bedroom to the kitchen in five seconds—it may take you a full two seconds to get from the living room to your refrigerator. My point: Small-apartment living makes it difficult to ever distance yourself from food—visually, physically, or mentally.

Before the pandemic, the close quarters of my apartment weren't an issue. Like many New Yorkers, I spent morning to night out of the apartment, and when I came home, my cozy space was comforting after the immense hustle and bustle of the Big Apple.

But after stay-at-home orders were issued, we all became confined in our homes and within walking distance of our kitchens. But in my apartment, I was literally working, sleeping, and living on top of food.

It didn't help that ABC set up my home studio within arm's reach of the kitchen (not that there were any other options, by the way!). While the spot looked great on live TV—and I'm thankful for the crew's expert eye—I could literally do a side bend and grab a cookie. Parked there for up to or more than thirteen hours a day, broadcasting for *Good Morning America, Nightline, World News Tonight,* breaking news, and special reports, I didn't have to think about what or when I was eating: I simply had to reach and chew. I hardly left my chair—which means I hardly left my kitchen.

Like many Americans, I also didn't have to make deliberate decisions about food anymore. Didn't have to decide what to order for lunch from my office anymore or what to bring home for dinner at night. I wasn't making decisions at the grocery store or area restaurants. The methodical routine of planning my meals, shopping for my meals, and going out for my meals was gone. Instead, food was there, next to me, around me, and available at all times. I felt like a lab rat in a cage: I just ate what was there.

The big X factor, however, was living with three kids in their early twenties—two who were college athletes and all three who were very fit and ate around the clock. Every two to three hours, they needed food. I'm not talking about some carrot sticks with hummus, either—a snack for these guys was a four-egg omelet with two different cheeses. Or they'd order pizza, tacos with chips and guac, or burritos the size of a football from my favorite Mexican restaurant. Since it was my apartment and I usually picked up the delivery tab, I often ate whatever they ordered, even though delicious New York pizza, chips, and burritos hardly fit into my usual low-carb lifestyle. But I was working so hard, it was a stressful time, and I felt like I deserved to eat whatever I wanted.

There was also the issue of my quarantine food. After the CDC recommended everyone stock up on enough groceries to stay at home for two weeks, I went online to buy canned sardines, crackers, and olive oil, along with an entire box of Lindt dark chocolate bars with salted caramel. If the world was coming to an end, I figured, I was at least going to enjoy it. But instead of savoring a square after dinner like I normally do, I began eating an entire bar nearly every day.

Two months into quarantine, I had gained almost five pounds. Moreover, I didn't feel good. I was tired, low energy, and achy, and had difficulty focusing and concentrating. I knew the reason: I was consuming sugar and carbs in quantities I don't normally ever do—and it was taking a toll on my physical and mental health.

When I started to feel terrible is when I woke up to what I was doing to my body. I literally sat myself down and talked to myself like I was one of my patients. I told myself that while it seemed like a good time to freak out about my diet, poor nutrition can be reversed by taking small steps, and those steps can add up to big results over time.

I looked at the two other aspects of my life—my physical activity levels and sleep hygiene—which, along with nutrition, make up what I call the *three pillars of good health*. My sleep was fine: I was averaging at least seven hours nightly because I knew I couldn't deliver the news on any less. But I wasn't moving because I wasn't leaving my apartment, which I knew wasn't helping my new diet.

I immediately started to add a little exercise (more on how to do this during a pandemic in chapter 5).

At the same time, I went back to the way of eating I knew had helped my body in the past. This was based on facts, not fads or fear: I had followed a low-carb diet for years and had evidence from my own experience that it helps me lose weight and feel my best. I cut out the pizza, chips, and other processed carbs and focused on consuming more lean protein, veggies, dairy, and healthy fats.

But I couldn't do it alone: Since my kids were part of the problem, I knew they also had to be part of the solution. I sat them down and explained I was changing my diet and needed their help—no more late-night pizza runs, quesadillas for dinner, or home-baked chocolate-chip cookies. I told them that this type of food wasn't great for their health either, no matter how much they exercised.

Within two weeks, I had turned it all around. I lost two pounds and regained my energy, optimism, and focus. Since then, I haven't gone back to stress eating or overeating, even as the crisis has continued and various stressful scenarios have developed. But I learned my lesson, and now I want to share with you how you can adapt and adopt that lesson, too, whether you have two or two hundred pounds to lose, or simply want to eat to optimize your health during a pandemic.

Here's the thing that's really important to recognize in our new normal: The pandemic has changed how we all eat. Everyone is cooking more, with surveys showing an unprecedented uptick in the percentage of Americans who now make their own meals. We're also snacking more because we're spending more time at home, whether we're working from home or simply not going out as often. Many people, like I was during initial lockdown orders, are also stress eating or overeating—habits that are difficult to drop even after life began to settle down again.

What's more, the pandemic has changed how we *should* eat.

Some people may need to eat less in our new normal because they're less active since they're not going to the gym or getting out of the house as often. Others may need to adjust their nutrition because they've gained weight, whether during initial lockdown orders or due to all the stress of the ongoing pandemic. Finally, we should all be eating different foods now to make sure we're doing everything possible to safeguard our health from the risk of infectious virus or other contagious illness.

In this chapter, I'll explain how the pandemic has changed how we all eat and what you can do about it to be healthier, avoid weight gain, or lose weight in our new normal. I'll also detail how the pandemic should change how we all eat, with the truth about eating to boost immunity and which foods and diet plans could protect you the most against COVID-19.

Finally, I'll explain how food can truly be thy medicine—or one of the contributing factors to the deterioration of your health. It's why I went back to school a few years ago to get my master's degree in nutrition. Since doctors aren't really taught how food can help or harm health in medical school, I wanted to learn how to help my patients and viewers eat to optimize well-being. And there's no time like a pandemic to view your refrigerator like a preview to your medicine cabinet. What you reach for in the fridge may very well determine what you eventually have to reach for in your pill closet.

HOW THE PANDEMIC HAS CHANGED AMERICA'S DIET

The coronavirus outbreak has changed what, how, or how much nearly every American eats. Before the pandemic, for example, restaurants made up 21 percent of our daily calories.[1] We now eat out a lot less and cook at home more often, with 60 percent of

Americans making more meals at home than they did before the outbreak.[2] In fact, 85 percent of all Americans have changed either what type of foods they eat or how they prepare it, according to a survey by the International Food Information Council.[3]

Many of our pandemic-induced dietary changes haven't been beneficial to our country's collective health. With millions working from home and others unemployed, Americans are eating more frequently, with surveys showing up to 76 percent of people now snack more often than they did before the outbreak.[4] We're also eating more in general, with overeating ranking as the third most common health concern caused by the pandemic, after lack of exercise and anxiety, according to one survey.[5]

What we're eating has also changed. In the first few months of the pandemic, sales of flour, sugar, pasta, salty snacks, alcohol, and ice cream shot through the roof. While we started cooking more, we also started baking more, as bread recipes went viral,[6] and we used our newfound kitchen habit to whip up dishes like pancake cereal, which dominated Instagram for weeks.[7] We're making fewer trips to the grocery store, where we find fewer choices on store shelves, as grocery stores look to avoid supply-chain problems.[8] We're also buying more frozen foods.

Perhaps the biggest change inherent in our new normal is that we're all eating more. The Quarantine 15 that many gained during initial lockdown orders has now turned into the Quarantine 30 for many. While reports vary, half of women and a quarter of all men say they gained weight during the pandemic, according to WebMD.[9] Another survey conducted by Nutrisystem discovered that 76 percent of respondents have gained up to sixteen pounds during the pandemic.[10] As reported in the *New York Times,* tailors in New York City say business is booming, with people bringing in pants, skirts, and dresses to be let out in order to accommodate expanding waist sizes.[11]

Weight gain and poor dietary habits prompted by the pandemic aren't easy to change and can persist for years, even after stay-at-home orders end. If you've started to use stress eating or overeating as a way to deal with anxiety or other emotions, it may be difficult to simply erase that coping mechanism from your survival plan. But there are ways to combat stress eating and turn a bad habit into an advantage (see page 91).

When Eating Less Isn't a Good Thing in Our New Normal

Not everyone has the luxury of eating all the salty snacks they want during a pandemic. The economic impact of the outbreak has caused or worsened food insecurity for millions of Americans. In New York City and other urban areas across the country, lines at food banks have stretched for blocks. Children who haven't been able to attend school have lost their one daily meal. And 60 percent more older adults now face food insecurity than they did in pre-pandemic times.[12]

These facts belie what's going on at many farms and food plants, where workers have destroyed crops, dumped milk, and smashed eggs. Without the same number of restaurants, hotels, schools, and stadiums to serve, suppliers say they've had no other choice but to toss perishable stock.

The pandemic has also exposed cracks in our food-supply chain. After outbreaks of COVID-19 hit several meat-packing plants, for example, the availability of meat shot down as the cost shot up. Panic buying, supplier disruption, and reduced transport options, among other problems, have also led to national shortages of dozens of food products.

The solutions to these issues are complex—and I certainly

don't have the answers. But I know that those who are lucky enough to have the problem of too much food should feel fortunate every day. Every meal I have, I am truly thankful to have food in the first place.

SIX RULES TO EAT RIGHT IN A PANDEMIC

Everything we do with our bodies during a pandemic can be critical to our overall health. But good nutrition may be one of the best protective measures we can take against the virus—and all other pathogens—short of wearing a mask and social distancing. Proper nutrition is not a guarantee you won't get sick with COVID-19, but it can reduce your risk of severe complications.

Part of the reason diet matters so much is that what we eat affects our waistline, and we already know that being overweight or obese is the biggest chronic risk factor for severe COVID-19 illness. Good nutrition can also prevent or help treat type 2 diabetes and high blood pressure, both of which are risk factors for the disease. Our diet can also hurt or help our immunity, making us more or less vulnerable to infection and illness.

But before we detail the best ways to eat, I want to bust some myths about immunity: There is no food or group of foods that will protect you against getting sick with the coronavirus. While hokey headlines have appeared, like "Eat to Beat Covid-19," these articles are based on fantasy, not fact. As a doctor who is also a nutritionist and believes in the power of food to prevent and treat disease, I haven't seen any evidence that a certain food or food in general will protect you against this virus or any other virus.

What's more, most research showing that specific foods may boost immunity are based on observation, not causation. What this means is that while scientists can observe that eating more oranges may improve immunity, most studies don't actually prove that eating oranges causes increased immunity. In other words, correlation does not imply causation. Otherwise, we might all think that the sales of chicken wings cause snowstorms because wing sales go up around big football games, which occur in the winter.

Understanding these facts, here are my six rules to eat right during a pandemic:

1. **Cut down on added sugar already.** If we've learned anything about diet, it's that added sugar is terrible for our bodies and brains. Added sugar, found in nearly all processed foods, appears to increase inflammation, with multiple studies suggesting that the more sugar we consume, the more inflammation we have. And the more inflammation we have, the more it weakens our immune systems.

   Sugar may be especially detrimental to those who contract COVID-19. While the data can change, current research shows that people with elevated blood-glucose levels are more prone to COVID-19 complications.[13] Studies have also found that having COVID-19 may increase a patient's blood-sugar levels, leading to worsening conditions.[14] Either way, the virus appears to "thrive in an environment of elevated blood glucose," according to the International Diabetes Federation.[15]

   How much is too much sugar? The American Heart Association and the World Health Organization recommend capping daily added sugar intake at 6 teaspoons or 25 grams for women, and at 9 teaspoons and 36 grams for men.[16] Since the average American consumes at least 18 teaspoons or 77 grams of sugar daily, almost everyone needs to make a significant adjustment.

   I recommend that you start by reading nutrition labels—look for the line "added sugar" on all packaged foods—to get an idea of just how much sugar you're currently consuming. Remember that surprising foods, even those considered "healthy," can be loaded with sugar, like ketchup, bread, salad dressing, yogurt, spaghetti sauce, smoothies, instant oatmeal, protein bars, and frozen meals. Aim to cut out processed foods or substitute with low-sugar brands. Sugar is an addiction, so cutting down can be difficult at first, but I promise that the suffering is brief. As is true with any addiction, you'll eventually find it easier to pass sugar up and you'll need less to satisfy your cravings.

Should You Worry About Sugar If You're Skinny?

Even if you don't have a weight problem, you should still avoid eating too much sweet stuff. Sugar doesn't care what size your jeans are—consuming too much will still increase inflammation, lower immunity, and boost your overall risk of illness. Don't confuse inner health with outer appearance: There are plenty of thin people who aren't metabolically healthy.

2. **Eat foods that come from a farm, not a lab.** You've likely heard this advice before, but subsisting off processed foods, as the majority of Americans do, harms your health by giving you lots of sugar, unhealthy fat, and food chemicals, and very little of the good fat, fiber, protein, and micronutrients we all need to thrive. The standard diet high in processed foods can impair your overall health and weaken your immune system.

3. **Consider a low-carb or keto diet.** Before I extoll the benefits of low-carb eating, it's important to realize that no large, de-

finitive study to date has shown that a low-carb or ketogenic diet is some silver bullet for COVID-19. There's also not an overwhelming amount of research to suggest either diet increases immunity.

In my opinion, the real reason to consider going low carb is the same that I outlined in chapter 1: Consuming a diet low in carbs and high in healthy fat and protein is one of the best ways to lose weight—and losing weight, if you're overweight or obese, is a surefire way to increase immunity. Following a low-carb or keto diet can also help lower blood-sugar levels, stave off diabetes, and help treat high blood pressure.

Despite what you may have seen on the Internet, you don't need to count fat or carb grams or prick your finger for a blood sample to make sure you're in ketosis—a state in which your body burns fat for fuel instead of carbs. Not only is it controversial whether everyday dieters can even reach ketosis,[17] but it's also nearly impossible to sustain these types of super restrictive diets for the weeks or months necessary to see results.

My advice: Make whole-grain carbs like quinoa, farro, rice, oats, and 100 percent whole wheat flour no more than a quarter of every meal. Cut down significantly on added sugar, eliminate soda, sweets, and other instant insulin boosters, and avoid adding sugar or artificial sweeteners to coffee, tea, etc.

4. **Eat your vitamin D.** If any foods have the power to boost immunity, it may be salmon, yogurt, white mushrooms, fortified milk, and other items rich in vitamin D. Studies now show that increased D can improve immune function, decrease inflammation, and even have antiviral effects—and their data is based on both association and causation.

There may be another reason to load up on more dietary D now: The people who have suffered the most with

COVID-19—elderly, obese, and black and brown people—
are more likely to have low vitamin D levels.[18]

For these reasons, I suggest increasing your D levels by
eating more foods high in the vitamin. Fatty fish like salmon
and mackerel is the best source, but if you don't like fish, you
can consider taking a vitamin D3 supplement, which is more
effective in raising nutrient levels than the other common
form, D2. The National Institutes of Health recommend
adults under age seventy get 600 IU of vitamin D daily—the
equivalent of more than three ounces of salmon or at least
five eight-ounce glasses of fortified milk per day.[19] If you're at
high risk for COVID-19, talk with your doctor about supple-
menting with higher doses of the vitamin.

5. **Limit your alcohol intake.** I love wine and tequila as much as
anyone else, but I try not to drink either too often, especially
during a pandemic, when booze can be especially deleterious
to our health. Despite the fact that many Americans started
drinking more alcohol during the outbreak, booze is the last
thing your body needs physically or mentally during a pandemic. Specific to COVID-19, excess alcohol consumption
can suppress your immune system, raise your blood pressure,
and boost blood-sugar levels.

6. **Keep up your cooking habit.** With restaurants shuttered and
some (unfounded) fears about the safety of takeout, millions
of Americans started cooking more at home, with surveys
estimating a 60 percent increase in the number of people
making homemade meals.[20] While not all pandemic-induced
dietary changes have been beneficial, this is one to sustain:
People who cook frequently at home are healthier and consume fewer calories than people who eat out more often, according to research.[21] For more on why to cook in our new
normal, turn to page 94.

EIGHT STEPS TO STOP STRESS EATING IN A PANDEMIC

For millions of Americans, the problem with the pandemic hasn't been what we're eating, but how much or how often we're eating. While I certainly made poor food choices at the beginning of the outbreak, what really impacted my waistline and mood was how much and how often I ate. My stress eating was partly due to proximity: I was home, within feet of the fridge and my kitchen cabinets all day, which is something I know many people in our new normal can relate to.

For others, stress eating has been born out of exactly that— stress—along with the feelings of loneliness, sadness, depression, and universal loss that we detailed in chapter 2. I get it: This is a really difficult time for us all, and it is human nature to try to self-soothe with food, especially sugary, high-carb items that can provide a momentary uptick in our mood. Many of us also physically want to fill up the loss with what we can put in our mouths. Unfortunately, any mood uptick we get with food is only momentary, while eating too much of anything—especially sugary, high-carb foods—can make us feel emptier in the end.

I want you to know that stress eating and overeating are really common problems—I talk with patients who suffer from them every day. But while they're common, they're not impossible to overcome. Here are eight ways I help my patients stop stress eating:

1. **Admit you have a problem.** It's just like every twelve-step self-help group: The first step to recovery is admitting that you have a problem. For me, step one to getting back on track was acknowledging that I had jumped the track in the first place. Recognizing that we have a problem can trigger the realization that something has to change, which is sometimes all we need to be able to begin to initiate that change.

2. **Adjust your input to your output.** If you're still eating like you're walking to work every morning or going to the gym after the office every night, it's time to rethink your consumption habits. If you're moving or exercising less because of the pandemic, you should also be eating less, plain and simple. This was my first mistake. In pre-pandemic times, I was out of my apartment twelve hours a day, seeing patients and walking around my office, walking to ABC or the store, and going to the gym most days of the week. But when I had to stop going to the gym and didn't step foot outside the tiny perimeter of my apartment, I still ate like I did before stay-at-home orders were issued. This was a big factor for me in weight gain and mood changes.

3. **Steer clear of peer pressure.** Families and roommates are all seeing a lot more of each other these days, with so many working or schooling from home. But just because your kid is eating cookies or your spouse is ordering pizza doesn't mean you need to indulge, too. Our eating behaviors are often influenced by those around us, but they don't have to be if we're aware of the effect. Stick to your own eating schedule and remember that what a fifteen-year-old teen can eat is different from what a thirty-year-old can eat, which is different from a sixty-year-old.

4. **Ask for support.** As New York governor Andrew Cuomo said, "It's not about me, it's about we." We're all in this together, and when you're hunkered down with your pandemic pod, your behavior doesn't just impact you—it impacts all of those around you. Whether you live with one person or five, it's okay to tell your squad that you're struggling with food and need their help. To soften the ask, make it about what's best for the team, not necessarily you, as having healthier food in the house will benefit everyone. If you have certain trigger

foods, ask that those be kept out of the house or limited to special occasions only.

5. **Find alternative paths of pleasure.** The pandemic has taken away many pleasurable activities, like dining out, hanging out with friends, going to shows or movies, traveling, shopping, and much more. While you may have turned to eating as a way to replace some lost pleasure, it's not a healthy coping mechanism, especially if you're overeating or indulging in high-calorie comfort food. Find something else that can give you pleasure whenever you find yourself tempted to use food for fun, like listening to music, watching a favorite show, or calling a friend.

6. **Remember that a pandemic lasts a lot longer than a bad breakup.** In pre-pandemic days, we typically turned to comfort foods after a bad breakup, a difficult day in the office, or some other unpleasant, isolated event. But these examples are short-lived and unique, not the norm and ongoing like a pandemic is. In other words, you can't self-soothe your way through a continuing health crisis. If you're using food to cope with feelings of fear, anxiety, loneliness, or even boredom, reach out to a therapist who can help you address those emotions without the help of a pint of ice cream or a plate of donuts.

7. **Acknowledge, then dismiss animal instincts.** Binge eating is a primal instinct. At the same time, the human brain has evolved significantly since the days when eating an entire beast by the fire was necessary for survival. Humans now have something called executive function, which helps us self-regulate, among other high-level cognitive skills. Self-control is what helps to distinguish us from animals. While animals will keep eating until there is no more food, humans know better. While it may be easy to believe that we deserve all the cookies we want during a pandemic, we can't do that if we

want to be happy and healthy. The next time you're tempted to overeat, recognize your animal instincts and choose to listen to your higher brain instead.

8. **Make the paradigm shift.** You can't keep doing what you're doing over and over again and expect different results. Realize that you have to make a paradigm shift about how you're eating and living in order to overhaul a bad habit and instigate change. You don't have to do everything at once or cut out five food groups to get that change, either. Remember that small steps can add up to huge results when you're consistent and patient.

WHY PANDEMIC COOKING IS A POWER PLAY

Before the pandemic, I avoided cooking as much as I do uncomfortable shoes. I disliked cooking so much that I'd volunteer to set the table, clear the table, and do all the dishes before raising my hand to make a meal. And . . . I wasn't good at cooking—at all. The times I'd tried to cook had produced only unappetizing results, and I thought I didn't have the patience or time for it.

But the pandemic reversed my lifelong unwillingness to cook in a matter of weeks, as it did for millions of other Americans. We are now reportedly cooking more as a country than we have in the last fifty years.[22] Supermarket executives say people are also taking on more complex cooking—a trend they say they don't see going away anytime soon.[23]

After New York City went into lockdown, I started cooking at home first out of convenience: With many takeout places closed and those open averaging more than the hour-plus it normally takes to get delivery in Manhattan, cooking was considerably easier and faster. But as I became more comfortable in the kitchen— and got a few glowing reviews from my kids, who clearly are easily impressed!—I started to enjoy the process of cooking, too. I also discovered that cooking gave me a sense of control at a time when everything felt out of control.

My gateway meal was a dish we featured on *Good Morning America:* baked peppers with ground turkey, mozzarella cheese, and marinara sauce. The recipe is from *Good Morning America* co-anchor Amy Robach's mother, Joanie Robach, who started an amazing recipe site called My Keto Home full of delicious, low-carb dishes. I never thought I could make something that looked and tasted so good, but it was super easy—and a massive ego booster after my kids told me the dish was the best thing ever. I started making my own modifications to the recipe while learning new ones.

I still cook today, as I've learned that there are some big benefits to the habit in our new normal. Here are reasons to keep up the cooking habit:

- **Cooking is cheaper.** Who doesn't love free money? When you cook at home, you save up to five times the amount of money you would spend when ordering from a restaurant, according to research.[24] While you may need to make an initial investment in pantry basics if you haven't cooked before, these items will pay off big time in your budget if you keep up the habit. Don't think you have to make only pasta or other inexpensive carbs to save money, either: Cooking with meat, seafood, and fresh vegetables and fruits also saves money, experts say.[25]

- **Cooking is more convenient.** This was the hook for me. Since my schedule is usually insane, I figured I didn't have time to cook before the pandemic. But when the outbreak hit, I realized it didn't take any longer to cook my meals than to order takeout, especially when you consider the wait time and the possible commute time to pick it up. You can make cooking even more convenient by learning a few fast go-to recipes, planning in advance, and shopping only once a week—which is a smart habit to adopt anyway during a pandemic.

- **Cooking is educational.** Cooking a meal is a lesson in itself for all ages and various subjects, including math, reading, physics, science, home economics, and nutrition. Plus, when you cook with kids, you're teaching them a life skill and fostering a new passion they'll hopefully sustain for life.
- **Cooking is therapy.** Before the pandemic, I assumed cooking was stressful, but I now know that nothing is further from the truth. Cooking has helped me slow down and take the time to enjoy a process, relaxing me in a way few other activities can. Like jogging, I now see cooking as a time to reflect and self-nurture. Making your own meals can also be a good distraction from whatever's going on in the world around you.
- **Cooking is fun—and one of the few social activities we have.** Not only is it relaxing, cooking is also fun—and can be even more enjoyable when you get others involved, especially now when we have fewer social options than we did before the pandemic. Cooking helps fill the void by offering a communal experience that can be different every night you try a new meal. In fact, trying new things like cooking can help couples stay more connected, according to the American Psychological Association.[26] Live alone? Cook with others and compare techniques and taste over Zoom, FaceTime, or Skype. I've even heard about people holding entire dinner parties over live video.
- **Cooking is control when the world feels out of control.** I gravitated to cooking because it lets me control something—when, what, and how much I ate—at a time when everything was out of my control. That uncertainty still exists, both in our personal lives and the world at large, and cooking can help provide a sense of normalcy and control. Cooking also produces immediate results that you can taste and touch, which can establish that you can do tangible, productive, and beneficial things to improve your life now.

- **Cooking is healthier.** I saved the best for last because you've heard it before: People who cook more frequently at home consume less sugar and fewer calories. Home chefs also have an easier time maintaining or losing weight: When you make your own meals, you control the ingredients and portion sizes rather than leaving it up to the whims of a restaurant chef. And whims can wreak havoc: Studies show that most restaurant dishes contain the number of calories we need in a single day, not a single meal,[27] while 92 percent of all restaurant meals exceed normal serving sizes.[28] Home-cooking also obviates the temptation even the healthiest eaters can feel when facing a menu of tempting options, no matter how many times they told themselves they'd stick to the salad.

Is Takeout Food Safe to Eat?

I've been asked this question on air countless times, and I think it's important to set the record straight: The coronavirus is a respiratory virus, and research shows that COVID-19 is spread through respiratory droplets and aerosolized particles, not through food or people touching food that's served to you. To worry if the coronavirus is hiding in takeout is an example of fear without facts. On the other hand, *E. coli*, salmonella, listeria, and other food-borne pathogens, which sicken thousands across the United States every year, can be lurking in foods, yet these outbreaks usually don't deter people from eating out.

During the early pandemic, I ordered takeout all the time. In fact, I made a conscientious effort to order food from local restaurants several times a week in order to support small businesses that I knew were struggling. My takeout bill went through the roof, and while I benefited, it was the least I could do to try to offset some of the risks essential restaurant workers exposed themselves and their families to.

HOW TO STOCK YOUR KITCHEN FOR ANY EMERGENCY

Coronavirus isn't the only threat that may interfere with your ability to go out and get food. It's helpful to know how to stock up for any kind of emergency, including a severe storm, food-supply disruption, widespread power outage, or flood. Don't wait until an emergency has already happened to prepare for it—you might not have the chance. Here are steps to get your kitchen emergency-ready:

Toss it out before it sickens someone. They lurk in nearly every kitchen cabinet: those foods far past their use-by or sell-by date or that will never be eaten by anyone in your house ever. Make room for essentials by tossing them. Throwing out expired foods also reduces the risk of eating something that may make you sick.

Think meals, not snacks. When lockdown orders went into effect early in the pandemic, sales of chips, pretzels, cookies, and other snack foods skyrocketed. While it's fine to have these on hand in an emergency, you can't eat chips and dip for dinner for two weeks. Before shopping, take the time to plan out actual meals that you can make if you have to shelter in place. Keep in mind that you may not have power, so include some canned and/or boxed items that don't need to be cooked.

Buy what you like, not what you see in movies. A big mistake a lot of people make is loading up on the foods they think they need in an emergency, not the ones they're most likely to eat. If you stock up on canned ham, for example, because you think that's what people should eat in an emergency, but you can't actually stand the taste, sheltering in place for two weeks is going to be more stressful than it already is. When the CDC warned Americans to prepare to stay at home for two weeks, I stocked up on sardines and Wasa crackers—two foods I love that I can easily turn into a sardine sandwich for dinner every night. But if I had to eat canned beans for two weeks, I'd be miserable and more anxious than I already may be if there are stay-at-home orders in place.

Don't turn an emergency into a personal health crisis. Stocking up on foods you like doesn't give you carte blanche to load up only on frozen pizza, Tater Tots, and Kool-Aid. Some comfort foods are fine, but an emergency, especially a viral outbreak, is not the time to play roulette with your health. Be sure your meal planning includes foods high in protein—think canned tuna or chicken, smoked salmon, beans, shelf-stable tofu, or frozen cuts of meat—along with vegetables (canned or frozen) and sources of healthy fat like olive oil, nuts, shredded coconut, and shelf-stable cheeses like Parmesan.

Remember liquids. If you don't drink tap water, load up on enough bottled water to make it for two weeks. And everyone should remember to include beverages they may want or need, like shelf-stable milk, juice, and/or powder-based drink mix.

Designate an emergency-food area. If you have enough space in your home, designate a kitchen cabinet or part of a closet as your emergency-food area. This way, no one in your household, including you, will dig into your emergency supplies simply because they're there. Your emergency cabinet or closet is also a good place to store extra medication and your first-aid kit (see page 74 on why you need both).

Don't panic buy. Panic buying became a problem in many areas of the United States in the early months of the pandemic, increasing food-supply chain disruptions and hurting many who suddenly couldn't find basic essentials. Panic buying can also harm you: Hoarding supplies increases anxiety levels and can lead to more compulsive behaviors.

And don't panic eat. Just because you have food doesn't mean you have to eat it. Unfortunately, though, panic buying often leads to panic eating. For these reasons, don't overstock and try to designate an emergency-food space if space allows. Remember that frozen and canned foods can keep for months or even years.

Everything about our new normal is different, including how we eat. Some of our new nutritional habits, like cooking more at home, are great for our overall health and well-being, but others, like stress eating and overeating, can be deleterious. You may not have realized how your eating patterns have changed as a result of the pandemic, but taking the time to self-evaluate and recognize the new habits you've adopted can help you keep the healthy ones and do away with those that may be bad for your health and waistline.

Similarly, it's also important to recognize that how we eat in the new normal *should* change. Some of us may need to consume less to compensate for lower activity rates and/or recent weight gain while everyone can stand to prioritize the low-sugar foods that can help safeguard our bodies in pandemic times. Remember, food is medicine, and with every bite, you have an opportunity to help nourish, protect, and treat your body.

CHAPTER 5

Exercise

If you're struggling to adapt to the new normal, know that everyone else is struggling, too—every single one of us. Some may be more confident in areas of the new normal, but no one has adapted to every aspect. No one has all the answers, and that includes me. So while I may have been able to navigate my way out of anxiety and stress eating, I haven't yet discovered how to enjoy exercise in the pandemic era.

This is not an insignificant development for two reasons. First, while fitness has always been vital to good health, it's become critical now as we face two pandemics—one physical, the other mental—in which exercise can play a key role in helping to prevent and treat adverse outcomes of both. Since I'm not as eager to work out in the pandemic era, my fitness has dropped, which has caused my physical and mental health to fall in many ways (e.g., my LDL has increased by eleven points over the past year, which I attribute solely to less exercise, and I'm not as cheerful as I used to be). That's not exactly ideal when there's an ongoing viral outbreak and another pandemic that may or may not be right around the corner. We need to be stronger now than ever before.

Second, the fact that I'm now struggling to enjoy exercise is like saying the Cookie Monster no longer likes chocolate-chip cookies. Exercise is integral to my identity; it's part of my DNA. I've been playing sports or working out in one way or another since I was seven. For about three decades up until the pandemic hit, I was at the gym up to six days a week, doing cardio, lifting weights, or some combination of both.

While it may sound crazy to those who don't like exercise—and no judgment, because I get that exercise isn't everyone's thing—I love the way working out makes me feel, physically, mentally, and emotionally. A good workout leaves me feeling fit, strong, confident, healthy, and powerful, like I can do anything I want with my body. Working out is my mental salve, what I do to stay optimistic, energetic, focused, clearheaded, and happy. Bad day? I go the gym to get over it. Long day? I hit the spin bike to reinvigorate. Great day? I lift weights or take a total body workout class to celebrate and reflect.

In other words, to me, working out in the gym is what traveling, watching football, playing sports, and a host of other hobbies, many also transformed by the pandemic, are to other people. Now that going to the gym or taking a fitness class is nothing like it used to be, I feel lost, if not a little depressed.

Despite these feelings, I've worked hard to try to find some joy outside the gym. I've done a hundred push-ups a day and held planks for minutes at a time after rediscovering the benefits of both in *The Self-Care Solution,* which I wrote before the pandemic. I've also tried doing other types of exercise at home, even though my apartment is small enough that when I roll out a yoga mat, only half fits on my carpet. When I was sitting all day to be on TV, I started wrapping resistance bands around my knees and doing hip abductor exercises in my chair.

What saved me, though, was rediscovering the joy of running outside. Usually, I don't jog anywhere other than a treadmill because I'm prone to Achilles tendinitis, and uneven surfaces, however slight, aggravate the injury. But desperate times call for desperate measures, and so far, while it's no gym substitute, I've learned to feel pretty good with running. I'm not at all where I want to be with exercise, but I'm doing a whole lot better than I was at the start of all this. In pandemic times, that counts as a victory, so I'll take it.

Today, I've come to recognize that I've suffered a loss in terms of working out: the loss of a passion that helped to define me. This loss is obviously nowhere near as devastating as the loss of a loved one, a job, or one's health, but it's still a loss nevertheless and one that's affected me greatly. If you've also lost a passion in the pandemic, it's important to recognize that so you can grieve it and move on.

But this chapter isn't about how to grieve for what we've lost in our new normal—you can learn more about that on page 44 in chapter 2. Instead, this chapter is about how and why to strive to make exercise part of your new normal at this point in time, when you're still laying the groundwork of what you want your new normal to look like and be. It's about how to find the time, space, and motivation to work out when both logistics and inspiration to exercise may be in short supply.

Everyone has a different story when it comes to exercise now. Some have started to work out for the first time in years because they finally found the time or flexibility with working from home or after losing their jobs. Others, on the other hand—and data shows this is the majority of Americans—have become less active or stayed sedentary as a result of the pandemic.

Today, many also don't want to use a gym or be around others breathing vigorously, whether inside or out. Others don't even have a gym to use after many closed permanently when lockdown orders were lifted. Some people have lost their fitness and can't find the energy to get it back. And of course there are also those who simply feel too overwhelmed by the uncertainty in our new normal to even consider trying to add in exercise, even though physical activity may be the best salve for fear of the unknown.

No matter your story, there are reasons why and ways how to make exercise part of your new narrative. We're all facing a new normal, and how we restructure that new normal is up to us. Whether exercise was an integral part of your life pre-pandemic or you're now just looking at ways to improve your situation, this moment presents an opportunity for exercise to help your well-being. If you can build a new reality that includes exercise, you'll be healthier, happier, and more resilient to whatever happens now and next in the world.

In this chapter, I'll share how exercise of any kind can become your secret weapon against infection, stress, and loneliness. Your physical condition and fitness have the potential to improve, even when other things feel as though they're deteriorating. And in an environment that often feels as though our freedom has been restricted, physical activity stands in the face of that, boldly reflecting that you still have the ability to move and be active whenever you want, even if it is in or around your home.

WHAT WE KNOW ABOUT EXERCISE IN OUR NEW NORMAL

While there are plenty of stories of people rediscovering exercise in the pandemic era, the coronavirus outbreak has caused most Americans to become less physically active. That's a troubling development, given that only 23 percent of adults before the pandemic met federal guidelines for the minimum amount of exercise: one hundred fifty minutes of moderate aerobic activity per week (or thirty minutes of cardio five days per week) or seventy-five minutes of vigorous activity, along with some type of muscle-strengthening activity twice a week.

New surveys and studies come out often, but reports largely show that those who exercised before the pandemic don't work out as often or have stopped altogether. One survey, for example, found a 32 percent plunge in physical activity since the outbreak began among those who exercise.[1] Step counts have also dropped, with data from fitness trackers showing up to a 50 percent dip in daily steps, as many have stopped walking around offices, across parking lots, in stores, or simply out the door.[2]

The problem with our national nose dive in activity is that less exercise has now become part of our new normal.[3] According to a survey by LIFEAID Beverage, one in four Americans who exercised at least twice per week before the pandemic aren't going back to the gym.[4] One in three say they will go less frequently than they did before.

Some have severed the gym because they're now using home exercise equipment that they purchased after fitness clubs shuttered at the beginning of the outbreak. Others have discovered alternatives like running outside or are doing at-home online classes because they are less expensive and more convenient or pose fewer safety concerns than a gym membership. In fact, 56 percent of Americans say they've found "more affordable" ways to work out without a gym since the pandemic began, according to a survey by TD Ameritrade.[5]

But not everyone who's given up on fitness clubs and classes has found another way to work out. Many have just stopped exercising altogether.

Of course, there are plenty of people who don't want to go to a gym or never did before the pandemic began. Many regular exercisers who worked out outside or played sports before the outbreak have been able to maintain those habits, with modifications. But for the most part, data shows that many who were regular exercisers in pre-coronavirus times are now exercising less—or not at all.

The reasons that many of us have lost our exercise mojo are manifold. Some gym users don't feel safe returning to clubs or classes where people are breathing heavily; others say it's a challenge or even impossible to wear a mask while exercising inside.[6] Safety concerns have also discouraged those who liked to play team sports or exercise outside where there are other people. What's more, many gyms have permanently closed as a result of the pandemic, leaving some without the option to work out inside even if they wanted or when bad weather prevents an outdoor sweat session.

But America's overriding inability to get back into an exercise groove in our new normal goes beyond logistics. After stay-at-home orders were issued, less or no exercise became a new routine for many—and that new routine has now become our new norm. Restarting an old routine after you've established a new one can be psychologically challenging, especially a routine, like exercise, that requires physical and mental energy under any circumstances.

There may also be a physical hurdle to resuming your exercise routine in our new normal. If you stopped working out for any period during the pandemic, like millions of Americans who were forced to quarantine at home, you've likely lost fitness, which makes getting back on the workout wagon that much more difficult.

Many of us also need inspiration to exercise, which has become particularly challenging to find in our new normal. It's not so easy anymore to socialize your workout and exercise with a friend, meet a personal trainer, take a fitness class in the same room as others, or play a team sport. If you're working out at home, transitioning from living, working, sleeping, or eating at home to exercising at home isn't easy. Some people have also lost their motivation to work out now that there are fewer weddings, reunions, swimsuit vacations, and other incentives to get and look fit. For the weekend warriors among us, there are also fewer races, games, and athletic events to train for.

Personally, I don't enjoy exercising alone. Working out with my two athletic kids, instructors, trainers, friends, or even alongside strangers at the gym motivates me and holds me accountable. Another mental hurdle for me that I know many others share: I associate exercise with the gym, and when I can't be inside a structured environment that includes cardio machines and weights, I feel less motivated because I believe I'm not making the same fitness gains, however erroneous that belief may be.

For those who didn't exercise before the pandemic began, our new normal hasn't exactly motivated the majority to pick up the habit. Still, there are inspirational stories of people who started exercising because they lost their jobs or began working from home and suddenly found the time or flexibility to make exercise a priority. Others have started exercising because it's one thing they can do after the pandemic curbed the ability to travel, socialize, eat out, and do other leisure activities with abandon.

Whatever group describes you, there's one thing we all have in common: The pandemic has changed how, where, when, and maybe even why we exercise. And those changes are likely here to stay.

WHY EXERCISE IS CRITICAL IN OUR NEW NORMAL

Doctors, researchers, and public health experts have said it for years, but the coronavirus pandemic drives home why we all need to exercise: No one knows when something like the coronavirus will threaten our well-being and make it that much more important to be as healthy as humanly possible.

Another way to think about it: If you're adamant about wearing a mask and social distancing—as you should be, since those are two of the most important ways to reduce infection risk—you should also be adamant about reducing your risk of severe illness from infection. And physical activity, along with good nutrition and proper sleep hygiene, is one of the best ways to accomplish that feat. While working out is no guarantee you won't get seriously sick with the coronavirus or any other illness—we reported on marathon runners who went to the ICU with the virus—regular physical activity can greatly improve your chances of staying healthy and fighting any disease, COVID-19 or otherwise.

What's more, consistent exercise has been shown to help prevent or treat overweight and obesity, type 2 diabetes, high blood pressure, and other comorbidities shown to increase the risk of severe COVID-19 complications. People who exercise may also have a lower risk of developing acute respiratory distress syndrome with COVID-19, one of the leading causes of death from the disease.[7]

While the data is weak on whether eating certain foods can definitively boost immunity (see page 86 for more), there's plenty of evidence to show that physical activity does bolster immune function.[8] The stronger your immune system, the less likely you are to contract certain infections and illnesses. Or if you do get sick, those who exercise have a better chance at fighting off infection or illness in many circumstances.

Our national need to be active in our new normal isn't just physical, of course. Exercise is also a mental necessity right now, as millions face anxiety, depression, loneliness, boredom, hopelessness, aimlessness, or uncertainty as a persistent fallout of the pandemic. If you don't think you suffer from any emotional hiccups as a result of the pandemic, I encourage you to reconsider: Almost all of us are dealing with some degree of uncertainty now, and whether you realize it or not, that uncertainty can take a toll on your mental and emotional health if you don't have a healthy outlet like exercise to help work through it.

How can exercise help ease uncertainty and other emotions triggered by the pandemic? In many ways. You likely already know about the runner's high that happens immediately after a good sweat session, but exercise's impact on mood lasts longer than this ephemeral elation. In fact, regular physical activity can work as well as prescription antidepressants in some cases to help improve depression,[9] while exercising for just five minutes can start to lower anxiety levels.[10] A recent study in animals also found that exercise may help people recover more easily from stressful situations, boosting our overall stress resilience.[11] Working out also significantly improves sleep quality and quantity (more about why you need both in chapter 6) and may help prevent and treat insomnia. Perhaps most impressively, exercise may help heal acute mental trauma or post-traumatic stress disorder (PTSD) by stimulating the nervous system to literally move past emotional immobilization.[12]

Personally, exercise has been integral to helping me get a grip on my emotions in our new normal. Whenever I feel like our world is coming undone or things feel uncertain, the fact that I can still go out and do something proactive to take control of my body and health is immensely empowering. The rhythmic movement of working out, whether I'm running, walking, or lifting weights, is also comforting, forcing me to stay in the moment as I put one foot (or arm) in front of the other. I also feel a sense of accomplishment after every workout, which has become increasingly important in our new normal when it feels like we don't have any control over anything that happens.

HOW TO EXERCISE IN OUR NEW NORMAL

There are two hurdles to exercising in our new normal. The first is logistics: where and how to get in a good workout, especially if the gym isn't an option for safety, financial, or practical reasons (or all three).

The second hurdle is how to motivate yourself to get moving—because motivating to exercise has been so arduous for me and many others in our new normal. In fact, I think the inspiration to get moving can matter as much as when, where, how, or how long you exercise. This is why I've devoted a whole section on how to motivate yourself to sweat when finding the energy to do nearly anything in the pandemic era can be difficult.

I understand that exercise isn't easy, which was true B.C. (before coronavirus), when many faced less stress and there were fewer hurdles in getting out for a run or to the gym. I have a lot of empathy for anyone who has struggled to find the motivation to work out, no matter what our world is going through. If you've tried to exercise many times in your life but can't seem to make it a habit, that's okay. You're certainly not alone. I want to encourage you to keep trying, though, even if you seem to fail at first. Every step you take toward exercise is literally a success, and the small efforts can add up over time and even produce amazing results. Sometimes getting hooked on exercise is just a matter of experimenting with different times, ways, places, and people to find what can sustain you.

We'll talk more about motivation in a moment, but first let's cover logistics of how to work out in our new normal so you know what, when, and where to do it.

Overcoming Hurdle #1: How and Where to Exercise

On ABC News, we told an incredible story of a young man from Ohio who built a home gym entirely out of wood in his parents' backyard after his local gym closed due to the coronavirus.[13] You should have seen this marvel. Zachary Skidmore's "lumber jacked gym" wasn't branches tied strategically to trees. The former U.S. Army police officer spent two weeks constructing seven total stations, including a functional bench press, a shoulder press, a cable-fly machine, and even a wooden-log treadmill.

Skidmore's story is amazing and inspiring, evinced by the fact his Facebook video showcasing his gym went viral. But most of us don't have the time, skills, space, tools, money, motivation, or even basic wherewithal to build a home gym out of anything, even store-bought equipment—and that's okay. You don't need to create a home gym or become a runner or cyclist to get active in our new normal. Here are some ideas:

» **Don't just try videos—*really* try videos.** Lots of people have a misperception about workout videos and that the only thing on YouTube is Richard Simmons–like 1980s-aerobics-era exercise. Not true. Tons of people have come up with super innovative ways to work out at home, whether you want to do cardio, strength training, high-intensity intervals, core work, Pilates, barre training, spinning, yoga, or some combination therein. Better yet, most videos on YouTube are free and don't require any equipment. The secret to success is experimentation. Finding the right exercise video can be like finding the perfect home or apartment: You'll probably have to look at lots before you discover what you like. For a live fitness-class experience, try live streaming a workout video on Instagram—many fitness coaches and athletes now offer live IG classes where you can watch in real time for free or a suggested donation.

» **Think outside the box—or the gym.** Long before fitness clubs and classes were staples on every city block, people got into amazing shape by playing sports—think tennis, golf, soccer, basketball, softball, horseback riding, ice skating, skiing, fly-fishing, and martial arts. You don't need to join a team or find a friend to play many of these, either: hit balls against a wall, shoot hoops at a local court, teach yourself karate, or get a pair of skates or cross-country skis and find a frozen pond or snowy field.

» **Discover the secret of steps.** For an entire month for my last book, *The Self-Care Solution,* I rigorously tracked and tried to increase the number of steps I took every day. What I learned in the process is that walking can be a great workout, even when you do it at sporadic intervals throughout the day. I suggest using a fitness tracker or your smartphone to record your steps so you can stay consistent and accountable. And don't forget about house walking, which has surged in popularity as an insanely easy technique to log steps when the weather's bad or you simply can't leave the house for one reason or another. To do it, set a timer or grab your phone with the goal of recording a certain number of steps and do laps around your house or apartment (added bonus if you can walk flights of stairs between laps).

» **Join the home equipment craze.** You don't have to build a home gym out of lumber—or even build a home gym at all. But a few strategic equipment purchases can make the difference between whether you stay sedentary in the pandemic era or get back in the habit. Home spin bikes, for example, are usually less expensive than other cardio equipment and have caster wheels so you can roll your bike in front of a TV or a set of windows, or outside on a smooth surface. Dumbbells, a Swiss ball, kettlebells, resistance bands, ab wheels, or a suspension training system like TRX are all relatively inexpensive, but can overhaul your ability to work out at home with a single purchase—which is why many of these items have sold out online and in stores since the pandemic began. Don't forget to check online classifieds for deals: There's been a big uptick in gym owners selling home-exercise equipment as clubs have closed.

» **Multitask—literally.** Why do a boring chore on its own when you can do a boring chore *and* work out? For example, I now cut the lawn at our family's farmhouse with a push mower, even though we own a riding mower, because pushing a heavy tractor around the backyard for an hour is a serious weight workout. In the city, I'll walk out of my way to get groceries at a store several blocks from my home so I have farther to carry the bags. In other words, sustained chores can be workouts if you attack them like workouts. Whatever household chore you have to do, whether it's to get groceries, garden, wash floors, paint walls, shovel snow, or give your bathroom a good scrubbing, there's a way to turn it into exercise if you intentionally try to do it with energy and vigor.

Don't forget about multitasking while at work. Try my trick of using resistance bands while seated at a desk or take calls while walking around your home. I also like to put my laptop on a kitchen counter so I stand more often instead of sitting all day.

» **Consider a different kind of personal trainer.** Personal trainers didn't vanish into thin air when the pandemic began. Many trainers now coach clients in parks or green spaces around cities. Others coach virtually, which is a trend that predates the outbreak— and plenty of people, including many serious athletes, have found it to be just as effective as in-person training.[14] How remote training works can vary from trainer to trainer and depends on whether you want a coach to help you start running or guide you through a weight workout. Compared to in-person training, remote coaching can be less expensive and more comprehensive and can include a group of people. Many remote trainers are also willing to answer questions by email or phone outside of dedicated sessions.

Overcoming Hurdle #2: How to Motivate Yourself to Exercise

Motivating to exercise has always been hard. But getting out the door these days seems to be more difficult than ever as we deal with safety concerns, fewer workout options and incentives, and increasing uncertainty. As a lifelong exercise enthusiast, I've found it particularly challenging to be inspired to work out amid our new normal. Here's what I've told myself to make exercising not only possible but also more enjoyable in the pandemic era:

» Treat your workout like a shower. You wouldn't voluntarily stop showering for a few days, would you? Exercise is the same— we need to do it on a near-daily basis to be our best selves, physically, mentally, and emotionally. For many, exercising in the new normal isn't as much fun or as exciting when we can't be in a gym, play a team sport, or take a group fitness class. But just like not every shower can be long and luxurious, not every workout will be amazing or even pleasant. If we did nothing but things that were pleasant and easy or felt good, we wouldn't get very far in life.

» Do it because you can. Lots of people can't exercise now because they're sick, disabled, or recovering from a debilitating disease or accident. If you can move your body in any way, be grateful for the gift, especially when so many are suffering. If exercise is something you can accomplish in these uncertain times, don't squander the opportunity: Take control of your health.

» Get technical. You don't have to work out with others to feel challenged. Social fitness apps like OnePeloton, Strava, Nike Run Club, MapMyWalk, and PumpUp offer online fitness communities that provide camaraderie, training tips, and inspiration while allowing you to track your workouts and compare your progress to that of others.

If social apps aren't your thing, you can also take advantage of technology's motivation muscle by using your smartphone, smartwatch, fitness tracker, or GPS device to record your training metrics, like distance, time, and heart rate. Use these numbers to challenge yourself during a sweat session or to create targeted workouts around pacing, heart rate, or other exercise stats.

» Post, scroll, repeat. One reason I like to post pics of my workouts on Instagram is that I receive so much support and encouragement from friends and followers whenever I do. I purposefully also check my IG feed for exercise inspiration. *GMA3* co-anchor and friend Amy Robach is the perfect example. She always posts pics of her runs or workout stats, and they inspire me to get out the door whenever I don't feel like it.

» **Write it on the wall.** I used this trick all the time in *The Self-Care Solution:* Writing your goals down on an old-fashioned wall or desk calendar where you can see them on a daily basis practically guarantees success. If you don't want to write down what you will do, write down what you've already done. Keeping a visual log of my past workouts always inspires me to continue the trajectory. Just one note: Make it print, not digital. While we all love our phones, the physical act of writing down what you've done or will do is satisfying and can help you succeed. You can also see your written goals or workout log regularly in lieu of having to think to open an app on your phone.

» **Do this and you won't need inspiration.** Olympic track and field runner Jim Ryun once said: *Motivation will get you started. The habit will keep you going.* In other words, once working out is part of your new normal, you won't need as much motivation to keep it up. But how do you turn exercise into a habit? Build it into your daily routine. Find a time in your schedule when exercise makes the most sense with work, family, and/or your natural energy levels (i.e., some of us are morning people; others are more eager to be active at night). No matter when you decide to exercise, treat your workout as sacred: Don't schedule anything else or get sidetracked by last-minute invites or events. Once it's part of your daily routine, you'll do it without even thinking about it—one reason why studies show people who work out at the same time every day are more committed to exercise than those who don't.

STAYING SAFE WHILE EXERCISING OUTSIDE

When it comes to coronavirus risk—or the risk of influenza, the measles, and some other contagious viruses—we know that outdoor activities are safer than indoor ones. So your risk of catching COVID-19 while exercising outdoors is far lower than if you work out inside a crowded gym or take a packed indoor group fitness class.

That said, there are precautions to consider when exercising outside. For starters, you need to wear a mask, unless you're exercising on a remote trail, isolated country road, empty beach, or other location where you won't encounter other people. I understand that exercising while wearing a mask can be uncomfortable—I do it every time I run—but infecting yourself or someone else with COVID-19 is far more unpleasant.

Many mistakenly believe they don't need to wear a mask when exercising because they're moving and passing people quickly. But it's actually even more imperative that we all wear masks while exercising. When we work out, we breathe more vigorously, and when we breathe more vigorously, we expel more respiratory droplets into the air. Unfortunately, we know that the virus can travel and linger in the air on those droplets. That means you need to wear a mask not only to contain your own droplets but also to prevent other people's droplets from reaching you, even if you're not right next to someone.

A good way to think about it is with cigarette smoke. You know how you can be a considerable distance from a smoker but still smell the smoke? Or walk into an area where someone was puffing several minutes prior and know it right away? The same is true of the virus, according to the latest aerosol science. And while it doesn't necessarily mean that these sparse viral particles can make us sick simply by being exposed to them, it does mean that you can easily run, walk, bike, or hike through someone else's droplets or vice versa, even when you think you aren't exposed—which makes wearing a mask essential.

If you wear a mask, do you have to stay (at least) six feet apart while exercising, too? Unfortunately, yes. I asked the same question to Dr. Anthony Fauci, the country's top infectious-disease doc, who told me that it's not one or the other—it's both.

One more myth to dispel: You don't have to worry if someone accidently gets sweat on you. There is zero evidence, at this time, that COVID-19 is transmitted through sweat—or blood, tears, semen, urine, or feces, for that matter. (Note: Although the virus has been detected in urine and feces of infected patients, detection does not necessarily mean it's infectious.)

All of this is not to discourage you from exercising outside. In fact, the risks associated with not exercising that you read about earlier in this chapter outweigh the risks of possible coronavirus exposure for most people.

No matter your new normal when it comes to exercise, whether you work out more, less, or not at all in these pandemic times, prioritizing fitness now is more important than ever. You don't have to go to a gym, spin class, or yoga studio to get fit. There are countless ways to exercise at home that can be just as effective and enjoyable. If you don't like what you're currently doing, experiment to find what can get you fired up to get fit. While some of us (I'm looking in the mirror) may have to dig deep to find extra sources of motivation to work out now, trying to make exercise part of your new normal will eventually turn the habit into what it should be for all of us: part of the normal, no matter whether that's old or new.

CHAPTER 6

Sleep

Sleep has a giant publicity problem in the United States. Most Americans believe that sleep is in some way a luxury, what we enjoy on the weekends or whenever our schedules allow. We see sleep as expendable, to be trimmed in, pared down, or obviated entirely when we have an early-morning meeting or young kids to contend with, a late-night project to finish, or a full season of *Shameless* to watch.

The pandemic has done nothing to encourage Americans to get back together with sleep—if anything, the outbreak has propelled us toward splitsville with our beloved slumber. According to surveys, the majority of Americans are now getting less sleep than before the pandemic began, with many experiencing disorders like insomnia and night terrors. In fact, one poll estimates that 98 percent of all Americans have developed new sleep problems since the pandemic began.[1]

Surprisingly, I'm part of this 98 percent. I say "surprisingly" not because I think I'm above disordered sleep—I'm clearly not—but for the last fifty years of my life, or up until the coronavirus hit,

I've always been a fantastic sleeper. During residency, for example, I could catnap while doctors were loudly discussing orders or test results in the next room or nurses were rushing patients down the hall. Today I can fall asleep almost on command, and it's a rare night when I toss and turn or wake for any other reason than to use the bathroom.

I'm a good sleeper in part because I've worked hard to be one, prioritizing getting an adequate night's sleep over other concerns. If I'm at an amazing party and having an incredible time, but have an early alarm the next day, I'll leave like a schoolgirl to go home and go to bed. If I have a flight to catch in the predawn hours, I'll crawl into bed before the sun sets. Even when I've really wanted to stay up an hour later for some reason or other, I'll make myself go to bed because I know sleep is more precious than anything I think I want or need to do. In other words, spending seven to eight hours in bed is non-negotiable for me.

My priorities didn't change when the pandemic hit. I started waking up at four A.M. to be on *Good Morning America* daily, but I also started going to bed at nine P.M. most nights. This schedule often required Herculean discipline, especially when I had just been on *World News Tonight with David Muir* and would have rather spent time unwinding by watching TV or calling my boyfriend than dutifully marching off to bed. But I usually refrained from doing either because I know that if I don't get enough sleep, I can't deliver the news with the same kind of insight and accuracy that viewers deserve. As a doctor, I also know that skimping on sleep, even if only for a night or two, opens the door for a host of health problems to come sauntering in, which is the last thing I or anyone else needs during a viral outbreak.

What changed for me during the pandemic wasn't the *quantity* of my sleep, but the *quality* of my sleep. While I was still getting seven to eight hours per night, I would wake up almost every morning feeling mentally exhausted, not rested or refreshed. The first time it happened, I chalked it up to a long day. But when it started to occur over and over again, with a "time to make the donuts" kind of regularity, I began to feel unsettled. I had never experienced anything like it before.

As a doctor, I often look at my own life like a medical detective: I always try to connect the dots between events or behaviors and signs and symptoms. But I didn't need to put my super sleuth hat on to decipher this one. When I took a moment to step back and analyze my life, all I saw was the pandemic: I was living in the pandemic, reporting on the pandemic, and helping care for my patients in the pandemic. And while I assumed the pandemic wasn't impacting my sleep like it was for others, I was having dreams about the virus almost every night. Some were nightmares, like the one I described in chapter 2 when I dreamed that I was intubated in the ICU with COVID-19. Most, however, were simply virus dreams—that I was reading about the virus, talking about the virus, thinking about the virus. I wasn't alone: The phenomenon of pandemic dreams has become a vivid reality for many Americans, interfering with the sleep quantity and/or quality of millions of people.

After I stopped to analyze what these dreams were and how they were affecting my sleep, I began to realize that I wasn't taking the time to download the uncertainty and stress that was happening all around me and inside my head. Instead, I was plowing forward without acknowledging my anxiety, forcing my mind to work overtime to try to subconsciously process the stress at night. As a result, my brain wasn't powering off, running on a 24/7 cycle of uncertainty and anxiety that manifested in a nightly picture show of pandemic dreams. No wonder I was waking up feeling mentally exhausted.

While I no longer suffer from pandemic dreams, I know that waking up in our new normal not feeling rested is an ongoing issue for many of my friends, patients, and social-media followers.

The problem may seem paradoxical because many have more time at home now, with fewer reasons to go out or get up early. But this lack of a consistent schedule is just one reason why many aren't getting the quantity or quality of sleep they need.

For this reason and several others, sleep may be more nuanced than other aspects of good health, especially in a time of crisis. For example, while you can eat less and move more in theory to see results, you can't always sleep more to improve your health. If good shut-eye was so simple, after all, we probably wouldn't have an almost $90 billion industry dedicated to sleep-promoting aids and technology.[2]

Because it isn't always possible to "see" the results of more sleep in the same way we can with other kinds of wellness, it may be easy to overlook how the new normal is impacting our sleep. But what's become even more clear to me now during the pandemic than ever before is that sleep is in desperate need of an image overhaul. There is nothing luxurious or expendable about sleep, no matter what may be occurring in the world. It's a medical necessity. Without sleep, human beings can't survive. Suboptimal sleep leads to a decline in physical and mental health in almost every possible way—many of those ways imperceivable to the patient because suboptimal sleep deludes the brain into thinking you're okay when you're not okay.

All this has been exacerbated by our new normal. Parents who have to stay up late to finish work for their jobs because they are busy caring for children during the day are missing out on critical sleep. Unemployed people who suffer from restlessness at night because they're worried about paying their bills aren't getting the shut-eye they need. Older Americans who are afraid of getting sick are tossing and turning or waking up too early after a sleepless night. The pandemic has given many people new reasons to lie in bed awake, to sacrifice sleep for something else, or to avoid it altogether. And whether we realize it or not, this altered sleep quality comes with a very real health cost.

In this chapter, I want to show you how and why nearly everyone's sleep has been impacted by our new normal. Sleep can be a huge window into our psychological and physical condition, and if we pay attention to the signals it sends us, we have the potential to address and respond to minor issues before they become major ones, just like taking care of fraying wires before they can cause a short circuit.

Even those who think they are getting an adequate amount of sleep (like I was) may not be getting the quality they need. We'll also talk about the widespread phenomenon of pandemic dreams and what experts whom I've interviewed say you can do to overcome the issue. Most important, I want to show you what you can do to sleep your best in our new normal, with tips on how to identify and treat the sleep issues that have now become common in the pandemic era.

HOW SLEEP HAS CHANGED IN THE PANDEMIC ERA

In medicine, we use the word *sequelae* to describe the chronic health problems often caused by a primary condition. Sequela means "sequel" in Latin and is easy to understand when you put it into context: Migraine headaches, for example, can be sequelae (sequels) of concussions; acid reflux can be a sequela of pregnancy. And in our new reality, sleep problems are sequelae of the coronavirus pandemic.

In my opinion, sleep problems were one of the first sequelae we experienced after the outbreak began—and they might be one of the last sequelae to dissipate if and when we adapt to our new normal. That's because sleep problems are like an obnoxious dinner guest who doesn't understand party etiquette: always the first to arrive and the last to leave. Sleep problems can be insidious and cyclical as well, causing a cascade of physical, mental, and emotional issues that make it even more difficult for the troubled sleeper to get the necessary shut-eye over time.

Given these facts, it's not surprising to learn that 98 percent of Americans say they've developed sleep problems since the pandemic began.[3] The majority of us are also going to sleep later and spending less time in bed, with 67 percent saying their sleep was healthier before the outbreak began.[4]

There are several factors for our collective tossing and turning, according to statistics. The primary one, however, is the stress and anxiety the coronavirus pandemic has caused or aggravated in the majority of Americans.[5] While anxiety levels may have redlined in the early days of the outbreak, when the virus was new and highly mysterious, the pandemic has proven that massive medical, social, and economic disruptions can happen at any time, flipping our sense of normalcy upside down at a moment's notice. This realization—that there's always a lurking and latent threat of significant status quo disruption—is momentous and may haunt us longer than the virus remains a danger to human health.

While fears over the virus may have subsided somewhat since the pandemic began, there is still a persistent and pervasive sense of uncertainty in our new normal. Many people don't know when they will find a job, return to an office, ride on an airplane, or take a vacation to a new city. We think twice about many things that used to be everyday activities, such as sending our kids to school, taking a subway or bus across town, or going out to a crowded restaurant or bar. Some are more anxious now about money, job security, or their children's future; others are continually concerned about elderly or sick relatives. What's more, everyone's daily habits have been upended, and no one can say for sure if and when we'll regain a sense of a regular routine.

Unfortunately, this overwhelming sense of uncertainty doesn't just dissipate after we drift off to sleep: The stress and anxiety can keep running through our brains, causing us to wake up at night and feel less rested when we get up the next day. Sleep problems caused by the pandemic are so pervasive, in fact, that sleep neurologists have coined the term *COVID-somnia* to refer to the surge in outbreak-related sleep issues.[6]

Even if you aren't aware of feeling a sense of uncertainty, there's still a part of our brains that knows when things aren't "normal" and may stay switched on while we sleep. For example, after I didn't see my boyfriend for the first two months of the outbreak, we were both struck by how well we slept together when we were finally able to meet again and share a bed. The improvement was massive and significant, which goes to show how the subconscious brain can be aware of what's happening when we sleep, even when we're not. If things are uncertain in your life, as they are in the world, your subconscious mind may be processing it even if your conscious mind isn't aware.

Other emotions in addition to anxiety and uncertainty are also fueling our inability to get a good night's sleep, including feelings of depression, loneliness, hopelessness, and aimlessness. The relationship between sleep and mental health is also mutually dependent, meaning inadequate sleep can also trigger or aggravate these emotions.

Another factor disrupting our sleep is the lack of a consistent daily routine. With millions working from home and others unemployed, many people can now go to bed and wake up whenever they want, trading in their pre-pandemic alarms and strict bedtimes for an erratic sleep schedule. While getting rid of your daily alarm may feel like freedom, it can actually create a new kind of cage, trapping you in the toil of being out of sync with your body's natural circadian rhythms.

Human beings are exquisitely conditioned to do certain activities at different times of the day, all based upon our circadian rhythms, which is a fancy word for the body's twenty-four-hour internal clock. When you disrupt your circadian rhythms and, say, eat at four in the morning or exercise at eleven at night, your body has a tough time adjusting, since it's conditioned to cuing your digestion or increasing your energy levels at certain times of the day. When it comes to sleep, going to bed and getting up at irregular hours makes it almost impossible for your body to settle into its circadian rhythms, which can cause you to experience difficulty falling asleep, staying asleep, and feeling rested when you wake up.

The pandemic has disrupted our circadian rhythms in myriad ways, as many of us wake up, work, eat, exercise, look at screens, socialize, and go to bed at different times of day than we did before the outbreak began—and oftentimes, at wildly different times now than we did the day before. That leaves our bodies and brains struggling to figure out if it's day or night or whether we should be preparing to go to sleep or amassing the energy to tackle a workout or work project.

We're also spending more time staring at our computers, smartphones, laptops, tablets, and TVs in the pandemic era. According to one survey, children in particular are spending 500 percent more time staring at technology.[7] Not only can this amount of screen time be detrimental to your mental health, increasing the risk of depression, anxiety, and loneliness, but exposure to the blue light emitted by screens also disrupts the body's natural production of the hormone melatonin, which helps regulate sleep.

Other factors that are part of our new normal are also affecting our sleep, including the fact we're drinking more alcohol. While booze may help you fall asleep more quickly, it's a proven sleep disrupter, shown to block rapid-eye movement (REM) sleep, reduce deep sleep, and cause you to wake up more often. What's more, we're getting less physical activity, which isn't exactly helping us drift into dreamland and stay there.

The Phenomenon of Pandemic Dreams

Millions of people say they've had highly vivid or unusual dreams since the pandemic began, with surveys estimating that 87 percent of all Americans have experienced the phenomenon now known as "pandemic dreams."[8] These dreams can be literal—you or someone you know gets sick with the virus—or metaphorical, like being chased by a mob or attacked by bugs. Pandemic dreams can also revolve around safety concerns such as being in crowds, wearing masks, or washing your hands. Some can even be pleasant, like finding a cure for the virus or seeing a loved one you haven't been able to visit in months. But what our pandemic dreams have in common, researchers say, is that they're preventing us from getting a good night's sleep and are proof we may need to do more to address our anxiety.

When I was having my own pandemic dreams, I interviewed one of the top experts on the phenomenon, Dr. Deidre Barrett, a psychology professor at Harvard Medical School and author of the book *Pandemic Dreams* (Oneiroi Press, 2020), for *Good Morning America*. She told me that many people are now able to recall their dreams because they're waking up more often during REM, which is the sleep stage when vivid dreaming is most likely to occur. And we're waking up more often because we're anxious about the pandemic to such a degree that it's manifesting in our subconscious thoughts.

This isn't the first time dream scientists like Barrett have seen an uptick in vivid, disruptive dreaming. After 9/11, for example, many Americans also reported having more intense or unusual dreams. And while these disturbing dreams can eventually subside on their own, you can take steps to limit them and mitigate their effect on your sleep.

WHY SLEEP IS MORE IMPORTANT IN OUR NEW NORMAL

I've told you about my three pillars of good health that form what I believe to be the bedrock of disease prevention and optimal well-being: nutrition, physical activity, and sleep. After reading the last two chapters, you already know how critical diet and exercise are to our physical and mental health in our new normal.

But in my triad of pillars, sleep may be the most vital component. If you're not getting adequate sleep, how well you eat or how much you exercise may not matter as much: Your body's ability to burn fat, build muscle, increase immune function, and reap all the other benefits of proper diet and exercise will be hampered. That's why the first question I always ask patients when they detail a troubling symptom or condition is "How are you sleeping?" Sleep is that powerful and that important.

In the pandemic era, sleep has become even more critical. Pandemics by nature are high-stakes times, both physically and mentally. Physically, you face the threat of a possibly deadly infection, in addition to all the other health risks that have always existed—everything from cancer to car accidents. Mentally, you're experiencing a level of anxiety and uncertainty that is lasting longer than the fallout from any other traumatic global event, such as a natural disaster. If you're not getting enough sleep in the new normal, you're stepping out into the battleground of our world already a little incapacitated, a bit exhausted, and less likely to succeed.

Analogies aside, the body needs adequate sleep to be able to ward off viral infection. That's why people who don't sleep enough are more likely to get sick after being exposed to viruses like the common cold.[9] In fact, research shows that those who average less than seven hours per night have three times the risk of infection from the common cold compared to those who get eight hours or more on a regular basis.[10] Sleep is so imperative to fighting off viral infections that not getting enough can even reduce the efficacy of vaccines, according to studies.[11]

Inadequate sleep also raises the risk of diabetes, high blood pressure, and other comorbidities for COVID-19. Poor sleep can also contribute to weight gain or make it more difficult to lose it. From a mental-health perspective, those who get less sleep are also more prone to developing or aggravating existing feelings of depression, anxiety, loneliness, and other unpleasant emotions.

The Real Risks of Too Much Sleep

It's not just sleeping too little that's become a problem in the pandemic era. Lots of people are now sleeping too much. While everyone has unique sleep requirements, most healthy adults shouldn't be averaging more than nine hours per night—a sign that something might be amiss with your physical or mental health.

Most of us associate getting too little sleep with health problems. But getting too much sleep, or more than nine hours per night, can increase your risk of the same ailments, including diabetes, high blood pressure, and the tendency to be overweight or obese. One study even found that sleeping too much may be worse for your overall health than sleeping too little.[12]

Similarly, spending too much time in bed can boost your risk of developing depression and other mood disorders. Getting too much sleep can also ironically make you feel more tired and lead to lower energy levels throughout the day.

HOW TO SLEEP BETTER IN CRISIS TIMES

You probably know by now that you can't just snap your fingers and make all the fears, anxieties, and worries that may be keeping you up at night go away. Similarly, you can't hit the eject button and end all the uncertainty that may be causing you to wake up feeling exhausted in the morning. What you can do, however, is take the specific steps outlined throughout this book to control your anxiety, lower your stress levels, and learn to cope better with the uncertainty that is now part of our new normal.

For many, controlling anxiety, lowering stress, and coping with uncertainty often means finding ways to comfort ourselves at night, whether it's keeping Netflix on autoplay, scrolling through social media in bed, or watching baking shows until all hours of the night. I've been guilty of doing all of these in our new normal to help take my mind off stressful things and find a little emotional solace. But the comfort you may feel with TV, social media, and other late-night distractions are only temporary—and unfortunately, these distractions can and do interfere with the ability to get to sleep and stay there. Remember that getting a full night's sleep can provide a longer-lasting, far more beneficial form of comfort, so try to minimize these distractions before bed.

As you work toward controlling the emotions that may be interfering with your sleep, there are distinct things you can do to improve both your slumber quantity and quality. Here are seven steps to sleep better in pandemic times:

1. **Practice Sleep Hygiene 101.** You might expect your car not to run well if you knew the oil was low, the timing belt was shot, or the tires weren't filled to full pressure. Similarly, if you know there's an obvious problem with your basic sleep hygiene, you shouldn't be surprised if you're unable to get a full eight hours or you wake up often feeling tired. Sleep hygiene is the environment and behaviors you adopt when you sleep and includes tips many of us have heard before, like making your bedroom dark, quiet, and cold before you go to bed (the ideal temp for sleeping is around 65 degrees Fahrenheit).[13] It also means taking certain steps like limiting your caffeine intake after lunch and pulling the plug on all screens at least one hour before bed.

2. **Take a tip from your dog, part I.** Your dog knows exactly what time breakfast should be every morning, which is why he'll whimper or slobber all over you if you happen to sleep past the hour. In pandemic times, take a page from Fido's playbook and get up at the same time every day. While being out of work or working from home has prompted many to jubilantly toss their morning alarms and sleep as late as they want, following an erratic sleep schedule is one of the worst things for sleep health and hygiene. Adopting a consistent sleep schedule in which you go to bed and wake up around the same time every day is imperative to restorative sleep, even if you average seven to eight hours per night.

   To adopt a consistent sleep schedule, set a bedtime alarm on your phone that reminds you when to power down at night, and a morning alarm seven to eight hours later. For those without a concrete reason to wake up, like work or school, alarms may feel arbitrary at first. But remember that the reason you're doing this isn't on a whim: You're resetting your internal clock in order to overhaul your sleep and improve your health in our new normal. Over time, you'll start to naturally feel tired around your set bedtime, sleep better throughout the night, and wake up without an alarm the next day, feeling more refreshed and ready to go.

3. **Take a tip from your dog, part II.** When you take your dog to the park and he runs around with all his canine buddies, do you see how he sleeps like a log after he finally settles down for the day? Yeah, well, humans are no different: Our bodies and brains often need to be tuckered out to sleep well. But the actual act of getting tuckered out is tricky these days when so many of us have less physical and mental stimulation than we did before the pandemic began. Most of us are exercising less frequently and not engaging as much with friends, colleagues, strangers, and the outside world as we did before the outbreak began.

   What to do? Two things: (1) Start exercising. For logistical tips and mental tricks on how to do this in the new normal, see chapter 5. (2) Get your mind active. Take on new projects at work or aggressively target a new job search. For mental stimulation outside work, join a book club (virtual or otherwise), learn a new language, start writing your great novel, pick up a challenging hobby like playing the guitar or chess, devour new books, and/or cook new recipes. (This last hobby can satisfy multiple healthy objectives in our new normal—see page 94 for more details.)

4. **Retrain your mind.** My sleep got disrupted after I started having pandemic dreams, which was happening because I wasn't downloading all the things happening around me and inside my head. And I wasn't downloading all the things happening around me and inside my head in part because I wasn't taking the time to meditate.

I've meditated on and off for years, and when I'm on, I feel less anxious, irritable, and stressed and more relaxed, mindful, and joyful. In the early pandemic days, I stopped meditating because I thought I didn't have the time since I was working fourteen to sixteen hours a day for TV while also seeing patients virtually whenever I had a quick break. This was a mistake. If I had taken just twenty minutes to meditate, I would have had fewer disruptive dreams (or none at all), improved my sleep quality, and increased my productivity and focus, all of which would have more than made up for the time.

Whether you have pandemic dreams or difficulty falling asleep, or just can't wake up feeling rested, I'd encourage you to try some form of meditation on a regular basis. In my experience, it's one of the best ways to quiet the mind. Studies show that mindful meditation—focusing on your breath and how you feel in the moment—can help treat insomnia and improve sleep quality and quantity while also reducing feelings of depression, anxiety, and loneliness.[14]

5. **Channel your inner Freud.** If you're having disruptive dreams, the ultimate solution is to try to reduce your anxiety and stress levels. While you try to do that, you can take other steps to mitigate the effects your dreams are having on your sleep. When I spoke with Harvard Medical School's Dr. Deidre Barrett about it, she suggested writing your dreams down with an old-fashioned pen and paper that you keep by your bedside so it's immediately handy when you wake up (but doesn't emit blue light like your phone, which will worsen your sleep problems). Keeping a dream diary can help you normalize the experience and identify patterns like whether your dreams make you feel scared, anxious, isolated, or uncertain.

   According to Barrett, you can also try to control your

dreams with a technique called dream incubation. To do this, think about what you want to dream about before you go to bed, whether that's basking in your favorite vacation spot, playing a sport with friends, or spending time with someone special. Visualize yourself doing the activity as you drift off to sleep; if helpful, you can also place a photo by your bedside that reminds you of the activity. Just believe that the technique will work. College students who practiced dream incubation in one of Barrett's studies dreamed about what they wanted to approximately 50 percent of the time; when they didn't have ideal dreams, they didn't remember what they dreamed about, which means those dreams weren't vivid or intense.[15]

6. **Channel your parents.** When you were growing up, your parents likely switched off the TV when it was time to go to bed. Well, today, it's time to channel that discipline and turn it inward because we're watching much more TV now than ever before—and it's sabotaging our sleep.

With safety concerns restricting many social outings and activities, TV viewership has shot up, with Americans now watching an average of eight more hours of TV per week (more than one hour per day) than they did in pre-pandemic times.[16] The majority of this increase is happening at night, with the biggest bump occurring between eleven P.M. and two A.M.[17]

Not surprisingly, more late-night TV has meant a lot less sleep for most Americans. According to one survey, 37 percent of people would rather watch Netflix than sleep during quarantine.[18]

But Netflix isn't the only sleep saboteur inside your small screen: TV news is also stealing many away from the shut-eye they need. Since the start of the pandemic, TV news consumption has increased by 64 percent.[19] While that might be okay if you love broadcast news like I do—it's my industry, after all—for others, consuming too much news has contributed to their anxiety and, consequently, their sleep problems. If you find yourself particularly stressed by what you see on the news, shut it off during the day and at night for a while, take a break, or reduce how much you are viewing.

7. **Rethink pills, even the ones you get at a health-food store.** Taking a prescription sleep drug like Ambien can be tempting when you're desperate to get a good night's sleep. But unless a medication is recommended by your doctor, I suggest you stick only to non-pharmacological solutions for your sleep problems. As a practicing physician, I know from experience that prescription sleep meds often cause more problems than they solve. Ironically, sleep drugs often lead to daytime drowsiness and lethargy, reversing the desired effects of a good night's sleep, and many aren't approved for long-term use, which can trigger dependency problems. There are also certain health risks with prolonged use of some sleep meds, including the increased risk of headaches, chronic fatigue, and digestive issues.[20] For this reason, prescription sleep medication should be used intermittently rather than habitually and indefinitely.

I also don't recommend trying supplements like melatonin, valerian, or CBD unless they're prescribed to you by a doctor. Unlike some physicians trained in traditional Western medicine, I believe dietary supplements can and do work—and because I believe they can work, I think they should be approached with the same caution as prescription drugs, if not more so, since supplements aren't regulated to the same extent as prescription meds. When you take a supplement without doctor supervision, you're also rolling the dice on what dosage you might need and whether it will interfere with any other medications you may take. For those who believe that supplements are harmless because they're allegedly all natural, I can list about two dozen "all-natural" things that aren't harmless, including cocaine, hemlock, tobacco, and opium poppy.

Sleep problems were prevalent long before the coronavirus pandemic began and will remain so for decades after this outbreak—and the next outbreak—ends. But just as the world around us influences how we eat, think, and play, it also shapes how we sleep, and recognizing which external factors might be interfering with your internal thoughts, emotions, and ability to sleep is key to adapting in our new normal.

The first step in this process is to acknowledge that the world we live in is different now and that your sleep has likely been impacted as a result. Once you start to recognize and normalize our new normal, you will be better able to take the steps necessary to stabilize your sleep, too. Doing this won't just improve your health and happiness, it can also help you view our new normal as a well-rested, well-refreshed person would: bright, in full color, and a hopeful place to be.

CHAPTER 7

Health Fears

Kristin Whitfield, seventy-one, is an extraordinary woman. Vivacious and outgoing, she's always been an intrepid adventurer, sailing big boats on Lake Huron during the week and dancing in jazz clubs with her friends on the weekends. She has traveled extensively, loves parties and meeting new people, and can mix martinis, shuck oysters, and bike with the best of them.

Of course, this was all before the pandemic hit. Immediately after the coronavirus outbreak began, Kristin had to shut down her life like millions of other Americans—and rightfully so. In her early seventies with a heart condition, she is at high risk for developing complications with the disease.

But after stay-at-home orders were lifted, Kristin wanted to restart life and began to plan a cross-country drive from her house in Michigan to her former home in Cape Cod. The only problem was that Kristen had now developed an acute fear of being inside anyplace other than her home, even if only for a few minutes. How would she make it all the way to Cape Cod? She vowed she wouldn't stop at any public restrooms during the drive, relieving herself instead on the side of the highway.

When I heard Kristin's story, I was extremely empathetic. She has every right to be concerned about catching COVID-19 and should be taking all necessary precautions to prevent infection. But those precautions had now crossed the line from necessary to extreme, and if she had reached the point of peeing on the side of the highway, the concerns she had about her risk of exposure to the virus had become overly anxious. And that anxiety could actually harm her health.

What if a car swerved and hit Kristen while she was stopped on the shoulder? That's a genuine threat, with 12 percent of all interstate highway deaths due to shoulder accidents.[1] Or what if she contracted Lyme disease—the most common vector-borne illness in the United States—by crouching in the woods to pee? Her trip took her through states with the highest density of deer ticks, which transmit the debilitating illness. Finally, what was all this anxiety doing for her heart condition? People who suffer from generalized anxiety disorder may have up to a 48 percent higher likelihood of dying of heart disease, according to studies.[2]

In my medical opinion, these risks outweighed the possible perils Kristin would have faced by using a public bathroom while wearing a mask—an endeavor that epidemiologists consider to be low to medium risk for catching COVID-19.[3]

Kristin wasn't someone I expected to develop irrational fears about her health: She is very outgoing and didn't have a history of anxiety or phobia. But pandemics can change people, including the fears we have about both our inner and outer worlds. And while her health concerns aren't as crippling as what many now face in our new normal, her story illustrates how health anxiety can manifest in subtle and oftentimes potentially harmful ways.

I want to be clear, though: Having some degree of fear or apprehension in our new normal is understandable, if not inevitable. Pandemics, by definition, are frightening times, and fear is a natural and primitive response. I'm a doctor, I understand disease pathology very well, and I deal with medical concerns every day as both a practicing physician and medical correspondent. But I'm not immune from feeling anxious about my own health from time to time (see page 37 in chapter 2 for my story).

But what's happening now for many isn't a passing flash of anxiety. It's an acute and lasting fear that's caused millions of people to become preoccupied with the virus or another medical concern onto which they've transferred their fears. This ongoing preoccupation can begin to interfere with your everyday behaviors and basic well-being, causing a level of anxiety that increases your risk of depression, loneliness, and isolation, along with many physical ailments like high blood pressure and irritable bowel syndrome. Health fears can also prompt some to make very unsafe decisions such as washing food in bleach or, like Kristin, going out of their way to avoid the virus only to expose themselves to other potentially harmful risks. Others have become so preoccupied that they have or will get the virus that they've lost relationships, career opportunities, and/or the ability to function in our new normal.

No matter how mild or acute your level of health anxiety may be, the good news is that the condition is largely treatable. You can learn to address your fears and enjoy life safely, even during a pandemic or similar health crisis. In this chapter, we'll look at what health anxiety is, how to identify if you have a problem, and how learning to think like a doctor can help you better adapt to our new normal.

I will carefully walk you through an explanation of why and how more is not better when it comes to anxiety about your individual health. I'll also share concepts behind some of the key medical mantras that I've learned in the twenty years I've been a doctor.

I've used them hundreds, if not thousands of times to help soothe many frightened and even panicked patients. I know these mantras helped them, and I believe they can help you, too.

ARE YOUR HEALTH FEARS ACTUALLY HARMING YOUR HEALTH?

In medicine, being overly fearful that you'll get sick or obsessing over your health is a condition known as health anxiety. Before the coronavirus outbreak began, researchers estimated up to 12 percent of all people suffered from this mental-health issue.[4] The pandemic, however, has significantly increased this statistic, according to at least one study published in *American Psychologist,* affecting people with no known previous history of anxiety or hypochondria.[5]

It's not difficult to understand why so many of us may now feel overly anxious about our health. As a world, we've watched as entire countries have shut down and our daily lives have been upended, all because the coronavirus has posed such a continual threat to our collective health. Many of the places we used to go for comfort and enjoyment like restaurants, gyms, movie theaters, and churches have become potentially unsafe to enter without a mask. We might not even ever shake hands again, according to the country's top infectious disease doctor, Dr. Anthony Fauci, because the virus is so highly transmissible.[6]

Just because you've agonized over the coronavirus, however, doesn't mean you have health anxiety. In fact, if you haven't been worried about COVID-19 at one time or another, I might argue that you're missing the body's natural fear response. Similarly, it's also entirely normal to feel pain or a troubling symptom and experience a momentary sense of panic that it could be something serious or spend a little too much time googling worst-case scenarios on the web. These are all natural reactions and responses.

But worrying about COVID-19, some other illness, or your health in general becomes detrimental when these occasional concerns turn into persistent anxieties. This can happen when the rational part of your brain becomes paralyzed by fear, allowing the irrational thoughts you may have about a certain illness, your body, or your overall health to take over and dictate your decisions, actions, and/or emotions. These fears can become crippling, leading to acute anxiety, depression, and other mental-health issues, and allow you to make choices that could harm your health in other ways. Health anxiety can even interfere with your ability to function around others or in the world at large.

It's important to know that this kind of health anxiety can happen to anyone at any time, even months or years after a traumatic event like a pandemic is over. The condition doesn't discriminate based on intelligence or education, and extremely smart people with multiple degrees behind their name can and do develop health anxiety. You also don't have to be older or at risk of serious COVID-19 complications to suffer. In fact, researchers saw a 133 percent increase in health anxiety in children and young people in the United Kingdom in 2020 compared to the year prior, according to a survey commissioned by the National Health Service.[7] Health anxiety can affect the mentally strong and emotionally resilient as well as those who might otherwise appear to be calm and content.

For example, I recently saw a twenty-four-year-old patient who was happily attending graduate school in Philadelphia when the outbreak began. As time went on, however, she developed so much anxiety about catching COVID-19 that she decided to leave school to move back home with her parents in New York City. While she hoped being ensconced in her childhood home would make her feel safer, her health anxiety didn't dissipate. When she saw me, she was acutely frightened of contracting the virus, even though New York City had one of the lowest transmission rates at the time, my medical practice was taking all the appropriate COVID-19 risk-reduction precautions, and she had no risk factors for serious complications from the disease.

How can you tell if you have health anxiety? Here are some questions to ask yourself to help determine if your health concerns may be causing you more harm than good:

» Are concerns about the virus or your general health causing you to feel isolated, depressed, lonely, or anxious?

» Are concerns about the virus or your general health interfering with your ability to work or perform other activities for your day-to-day livelihood?

» Are concerns about the virus or your general health interfering with your relationships or ability to give or receive love?

» Are you taking risks you wouldn't have before the pandemic to avoid possible exposure to the virus?

» Are you not leaving your home because you're concerned about the virus (barring stay-at-home orders or the need to self-quarantine)?

» Do you spend an obsessive amount of time sterilizing your body, home, or other surroundings?

» Do you have no signs of infection or illness but constantly worry you have COVID-19 or another medical condition?

» Do you spend an obsessive amount of time googling the virus or other medical conditions?

» Are your concerns about the virus or general health interfering with your ability to sleep or eat?

» Do you find yourself worrying about the virus or your general health multiple times per day?

» Have any of your friends or family told you that your fears or safety precautions are extreme?

If you answered yes to one or more of these questions, it is possible that you may be suffering from health anxiety. Keep reading to find out ways to help ease this anxiety and how to start thinking like a doctor to navigate our new normal healthfully, happily, and safely.

When to Seek Help

If you answered yes to multiple questions in the preceding list, you may be suffering from acute hypochondriasis. Two-thirds of all people diagnosed with hypochondriasis also have a co-existing psychiatric disorder like depression, panic disorder, or obsessive-compulsive disorder (OCD), all of which are serious conditions that may require targeted treatment.[8] If you or those around you are concerned about your health anxiety, seek professional help immediately from a psychologist, psychiatrist, or other mental-health professional.

SIX STEPS TO HELP EASE HEALTH ANXIETY

During a major health crisis like a pandemic, it can be easy to feel like you need to stop living a normal life in order to keep living any kind of life in the future. But that's just not true. You don't have to live in fear in order to protect yourself against the coronavirus or any other medical condition. Here are six steps you can take now to try to mitigate your health fears. The first five are relatively straightforward; the last step takes some extra intel, which you'll find detailed in the remainder of this chapter.

1. **Recognize and normalize the issue.** You've come across this advice in earlier chapters, but there's a reason I keep repeating it: In our new normal, it's critical to recognize the hurdles we face in order to get over them and keep moving forward, and the first step to overcoming health anxiety is to admit that it exists in the first place. There's no shame or embarrassment when you do this, either: Health anxiety is a common occurrence and not a reflection of your intelligence, education, sophistication, mental strength, or emotional resilience.

   Acknowledging that you have health anxiety can also help normalize the problem. When you tell yourself (and others) that you're suffering, it allows you to accept your fears and start to see them as common and commonplace instead of abnormal and scary.

2. **You don't have to tell yourself it's in your head.** Your fears are real in the sense that they're really happening to you. And sometimes, very real fears can create symptoms like difficulty breathing, chest tightness, headaches, fatigue, body aches, and nausea, all of which are also symptoms of COVID-19, among other things. Remember the story on page 41 about my colleagues who have called me because they had chest tightness and thought they had COVID-19? That symptom was due to anxiety, not the virus.

   The next time you find yourself zeroing in on perceived symptoms—or taking excessive precautions like over-sanitizing or convincing yourself you will get sick—think instead about what you're missing by obsessing over your health, including time with family or friends, the opportunity to get ahead at your job, or the chance to practice self-care.

3. **Consider CBT.** According to researchers and leading mental-health organizations, cognitive behavioral therapy (CBT) is one of the most effective treatments for health anxiety.[9] In fact, one study found that CBT doubled the likelihood of treating health anxiety over standard care.[10]

   CBT targets negative thought patterns as the root of our emotions and behavior rather than fingering a certain situation as the cause. For example, not everyone has developed health anxiety as a result of the pandemic. CBT can help you manage irrational thoughts and behaviors by guiding you to react to a situation without fear.

4. **Take a vacation from Google Search, social media, and even the news.** It's easy for anyone who spends enough time online looking up medical conditions to develop unhealthy fears about their body or diseases—it's why many medical school students think they have whatever ailment they're studying at the time. If you're suffering with fears about the virus or your general health, take a break from Google and looking up anything related to COVID-19 and/or other medical conditions.

   Similarly, spending less time on social media or watching the news can also help limit anxiety. Remember that some media outlets sensationalize topics—*if it bleeds, it leads,* as the saying goes—and stories of healthy people getting seriously sick with COVID-19 are the rarity, not the norm.

5. **Remember that common things occur commonly.** Many people with health anxiety tend to worry about medical issues for which they have a relatively low risk. For example, many Americans are now more fearful of COVID-19 than heart disease, even though their risk of dying from the virus

is extremely low, while their risk of death from heart disease is one in seven. These statistics shouldn't cause you start to worrying about heart disease, but it's important to keep your health in perspective as well as in an accurate medical context.

6. **Choose facts over fear.** As you know from chapter 2, this has been my maxim throughout the pandemic and ultimately what helped me get over my anxiety. Choosing facts over fear puts you in the driver's seat of your own emotions. Doctors do it every day in order to deal with harrowing health emergencies and to make medical decisions. If you can learn to think like a doctor, you can stay calm and collected about certain risks while minimizing the harms that health anxiety can have on your physical and mental well-being.

Don't Be a Health Hot Dog

Some people don't have any health concerns as a result of our new normal. They realize the risks of the virus and take necessary precautions while remaining calm and informed about the threat the pandemic poses.

Other people, however, have taken it to the opposite end of the extreme and are what I call health hot dogs: They think they're invulnerable or invincible to the virus and flout safety recommendations or medical guidelines as a result. Many young people have adopted this attitude, assuming they can't get sick and not wearing masks and/or social distancing as a result—only to come down with COVID-19 and admit that they should have taken safety measures. Older people can be health hot dogs, too, oftentimes because they're unwilling to accept the increasing vulnerability of their age or believe they've out-lived enough health hazards over the years and are somehow indestructible now.[11]

If you picked up this book, you're probably not a health hot dog. But if you know someone who is, I would encourage you to tell them what I've said on air many times: It only has to hap-pen once. And I know from experience that infectious diseases don't care how old you are or how many other viruses, patho-gens, or similar medical perils you've already survived to make you seriously ill now.

But there's a much greater problem with being a health hot dog in our new normal—or during any pandemic, for that mat-ter. While it's a free country and it may be okay for you to roll the dice on your own survival, it's not okay for you to endanger the lives of others. A contagious disease is not like cancer, heart disease, or other chronic illnesses: The choices you make about your own body and health can affect other people's survival.

THINK LIKE A DOCTOR— NOW MORE THAN EVER

Doctors don't use emotions to make medical decisions. We don't decide to operate because we're frightened by a disease or pre-scribe a drug because we're afraid of what will happen if we don't. Instead, we rely on facts and use evidence-based medicine, peer-reviewed published literature, patient data, population research, and known medical probability to make informed decisions about someone else's health.

Choosing evidence over emotion like a doctor can allow you to do something I talked about in the introduction: adopt a big-picture perspective of what's going on. If you look up the statis-tics for COVID-19, for example, you'll discover that your odds of getting seriously sick or dying from the disease are very low. For example, in mid-August of 2020, there were more than 5 million confirmed cases of COVID-19 and 170,000 deaths in the United States recorded since the outbreak began.[12] There are more than 300 million people living in the United States. Remember, these are facts, not fears or opinions.

Now let's put these facts into perspective. According to the National Safety Council, your odds of getting into a fatal car crash in the United States in August of 2020 were 1 in 114.[13] Your odds of dying from a fall in the United States during the same time were 1 in 127. These odds were greater than your chances of contracting COVID-19, but you likely never thought twice about getting inside a car or walking up or down stairs. And while your odds of a deadly car crash or fatal fall were higher than your chances of dying from COVID-19 *if* you became infected, there's no possibility of a vaccine for vehicular accidents or falls, and the risk of dying from either will last far longer than any pandemic. This is why perspective is so important, which facts can help provide.

One important note: Calculating your health risk doesn't necessitate spending a lot of time online doing open-ended Google searches or reading every article you come across. We'll discuss how to find reliable medical information in more detail in chapter 8, but in short, be selective about where you get your data just like a doctor would, relying primarily on large credible health agencies like the National Safety Council, the CDC, the National Institutes of Health (NIH), and the World Health Organization (WHO).

Thinking like a doctor also means educating yourself on a disease or health concern. "Fear springs from ignorance," as Ralph Waldo Emerson said,[14] and the best way to fight ignorance—and thereby fear—is with knowledge.

In the instance of an infectious illness like COVID-19, you don't need to take a crash course in epidemiology or be able to polish off articles on immunology or infectious diseases in *The Lancet* with

100 percent comprehension—you just need a basic understanding of how pathogens work. This understanding will help you better navigate any outbreak or pandemic, because while the research on infectious diseases can change daily, basic pathology doesn't.

Let's start with microbiology 101. What we know about the coronavirus is that it's part of a family of common viruses that affect both animals and humans. Viruses like the coronavirus are one type of microorganism that can cause infectious diseases; bacteria, parasites, and fungi can also infect humans and lead to illness. But these microbes all act differently in the body, and we can't compare a bacterial infection (like strep throat or a urinary tract infection) to a parasitic infection (like head lice or giardia), to a fungal infection (like athlete's foot or ringworm), or to a viral infection (like COVID-19 or HIV).

There are more viruses than stars in the known universe, with trillions in our air at any given time. In fact, an estimated 800 million rain on every square meter of Earth every day, according to research.[15] Hundreds of virus families can infect humans, and some can even play a protective role in the body. You actually have about 38 trillion virus cells in your body right now as you're reading this.[16]

And viruses that harm humans aren't all alike—there are different means of transmission and illness associated with each. Some viruses, like HIV, are spread through sexual contact, while others, like West Nile virus, are spread through insects. Foodborne viruses like hepatitis A are transmitted primarily through food and water contaminated with feces. Respiratory viruses like the coronavirus and influenza are transmitted mainly through the air and infect the respiratory tract.

Specific to COVID-19, the virus is spread primarily through respiratory droplets, which are microscopic globules made up of saliva, mucus, and other material expelled from the lungs and nose when people breathe, talk, laugh, sing, sneeze, and cough. These droplets can linger in the air or attach to surfaces and survive for several hours after being expelled. The disease can also be spread through aerosolized particles. The difference between transmission through aerosolized particles and respiratory droplets is that the former can travel farther in the air, are smaller in size, and linger for a longer period of time, which is why they're considered "airborne" or aerosolized. Droplets, on the other hand, are larger, travel a shorter distance from the source, and tend to fall to the ground more quickly, meaning the spread is more likely to occur through closer contact.

People become infected with the coronavirus when they breathe in respiratory droplets or aerosolized particles that contain the virus. But contact with viral particles doesn't guarantee infection: People need to be exposed to the infectious dose, or the amount of a virus needed to cause disease, in order for the coronavirus to multiply inside the body and cause COVID-19. While the science changes daily, we don't know the infectious dose necessary to cause COVID-19.

What we do know, as of September 2020, is that the *primary* mode of COVID-19 transmission is through direct or close contact with an infected person, which is defined as less than six feet by the CDC.[17] The at-least-six-feet measurement is not written in stone, however, and may evolve to a greater distance as research progresses. However, according to the CDC, "the more closely a person interacts with others and the longer that interaction, the higher the risk of COVID-19 spread."[18]

The coronavirus can also be spread through airborne transmission, which occurs when viral particles linger in the air after being expelled by an infected individual. According to the WHO, airborne transmission of COVID-19 is most likely to occur in indoor places that are crowded or inadequately ventilated, such as bars, nightclubs, and churches, where people may also be talking loudly or singing, thereby expelling more viral particles.

What's less likely is contracting the disease through what scientists call fomite transmission, which is a fancy term for viral spread through a contaminated surface. To date, there are no documented cases of COVID-19 infection through touching a contaminated surface and then touching the mouth or nose, although the CDC and WHO both acknowledge the possibility.[19] There is also no evidence to show that the coronavirus can be spread through blood, urine, feces, tears, semen, or sweat.

Why is all this information important if you're not an epidemiologist? I believe that learning about a disease saps the fear from it and turns what might feel like a frightening mystery into a set of scientific circumstances. Doctors aren't afraid of diseases, even relatively new ones like COVID-19, because we've spent years studying basic pathology. You don't need to spend years—you just need a few minutes of good solid research. Reread the last several pages and look up anything you don't know or which interests you.

I get that some things are scary, but knowledge really is power when it comes to our health. We're not paralyzed by fears over the flu—another virus, by the way—because we know so much about it and we've normalized it. You can normalize COVID-19, too, by learning everything you can about it. I've heard this from patients and viewers alike: The more they learn about the disease, the less frightened they are by it.

Believe in Your Body's Immune System

If you're scared of COVID-19, I suggest you try to turn your fear into faith—for your body's immune system. As a doctor, I know that the human immune system is nothing short of miraculous. It's one of the most complex biological systems in the world and is said to be more powerful than any drug invented to date.[20] Since you were born, your immune system has been working 24/7 to protect you from millions of microorganisms, fighting off hundreds of harmful microbes every day without your knowledge. Believing in the power of your immune system and that it's doing everything it can to keep you safe in our new normal can boost mental health while improving your physical well-being: Studies show that being optimistic and hopeful about your medical outcomes may increase immune function.[21]

WHY MORE ISN'T ALWAYS BETTER

When you're worried about your health, it's only natural to want to take every precaution possible to try to ease your anxiety. But not all precautions are necessary or even effective in preventing infection or illness, and adopting certain behaviors in the presence of some pathogens can even increase your risk of getting sick.

In the instance of COVID-19, we know that precautions like wearing a mask, keeping at least six feet from others (farther away is likely even safer), washing your hands frequently, and avoiding crowded spaces are evidence-based, effective, and even imperative ways to reduce your risk of infection. All of these measures have a low risk and very high benefit. But other popular precautions, like wearing gloves, don't have the science to show they help lower the risk of infection and may even boost your chances of contracting COVID-19.

Here are some common precautions to avoid, all of which can help you live more safely and with less anxiety in our normal:

» **Don't wear gloves.** I've talked about this on air multiple times because it's a really important concept: Unless you're trained in sterile technique and concepts of cross-contamination, most people should not wear gloves to protect themselves against COVID-19. If you do, you may be increasing your risk of exposure to the virus.

Gloves provide people with a false sense of protection. When you wear gloves in a public place, you likely touch more than you would with your bare hands, including doorknobs, store products, your mask, your cellphone, your glasses, your credit cards, your handbag, etcetera. When you touch nonsterile items with sterile gloves, you cross-contaminate everything and spread more germs by touching more things.

Doctors, on the other hand, only touch a patient and those items we know to be sterile whenever we wear gloves. As soon as we touch something that isn't sterile, we recognize that our gloves have been contaminated and will need to be replaced immediately to avoid germ transmission and exposure.

The layperson doesn't know this. Instead, when you wear gloves in public, you go home, remove them, and (hopefully) wash your hands. But the moment you use your clean hands to take off your mask or pick up your phone, glasses, purse, or anything else contaminated by your gloves, you're exposing yourself to possible pathogens—and probably more microbes than if you had touched these items with bare hands.

Another reason not to wear gloves is that there's no documented cases of COVID-19 being spread through contaminated surfaces—again, it's a respiratory virus that is spread primarily through respiratory droplets and aerosol particles. If you're wearing gloves but not a mask—or not a mask that covers your mouth *and* nose—you're doing yourself a serious disservice.

Safety Tips from the OR

As an OB-GYN, I have spent a lot of time in the operating room, performing surgeries like hysterectomies and C-sections. This means I know how to stay safe in the presence of potentially deadly pathogens. You can increase your awareness, too, by learning about the basic principles of operating room safety.

First, the steps doctors take to ensure sterility in the OR are primarily done to protect the patient, not the doctors or nurses in the room. The main reason surgeons wear masks, for example, is to prevent our germs from contaminating the patient, not to prevent *our* exposure to possible pathogens.

Doctors wear gloves in the OR to protect the patient, not ourselves, but as soon we put them on, we don't touch *anything* that's not sterile other than a patient's body. If we do touch something, we know our gloves are contaminated and thereby unsafe. This is why surgeons don't bring gloved hands below their torso—it's a training technique we learn so that it's ingrained not to touch anything while wearing gloves. We're so schooled in this technique that we'll ask a circulating nurse in the OR to scratch an itch, push up our glasses, or fix our masks for us.

The same applies to clean hands: Contrary to what you see on *Grey's Anatomy*, doctors wash their hands before surgery with their masks covering their nose and mouth, not around their necks. Otherwise, we'd have to touch an unsterile mask after we've washed our hands, which would contaminate our hands.

Finally, surgeons don't wear every piece of protective gear available to them just because they can. For example, I could wear a sterile hood or white-paper hazmat suit like those now popular with anxious air travelers whenever I operated on a patient, but doing so would be uncomfortable, restrict movement, and possibly increase the risk of cross-contamination.[22]

» **Don't sanitize your food.** The coronavirus is transmitted through respiratory droplets or aerosolized particles, not food or drink. It is highly unlikely and undocumented to date that you can contract the virus because someone touched the sandwich you ate or breathed in the vicinity of your French fries. Despite these facts, some people have mistakenly assumed that if hand sanitizer is good for their hands, it must be good for other organic material like food. Not true: Hand sanitizer can be poisonous and even fatal when ingested, which has sadly already happened to several Americans who've died after eating sanitized food.

» **Don't sanitize your groceries.** The CDC never recommended at any point in time that the general public sanitize their groceries, and there's no documented cases of anyone contracting the virus from food containers or packaging. But wiping down your groceries with bleach can harm your health in other ways. Studies show the fumes emitted by bleach can trigger symptoms similar to COVID-19, like shortness of breath and coughing; can acerbate asthma and other lung conditions; and can boost the risk of serious health problems.[23] In addition, using bleach on food containers increases the likelihood of contaminating food with the toxic chemical, which can burn skin and is poisonous when ingested.

» **Don't wash and sanitize at the same time.** Many viewers have asked me if it's best to wash your hands and then use hand sanitizer as an extra safety measure. Millions of Americans already do this, but the reality is that you actually may be harming your health by doing so.

Hot water, soap, and hand sanitizer dry out skin, stripping essential oils and reducing its natural moisture barrier. When you wash and sanitize consecutively, you give your skin a double-drying treatment, leaving your hands more prone to developing microscopic cuts. You won't be able to see or feel these tiny cuts, but they provide a fantastic portal for infectious microbes, including staph, which can cause you to experience a rash, fever, swelling, and tenderness. You can also contract MRSA, a type of staph infection that can cause serious complications. This is where perspective can help with health anxiety: If you're washing and sanitizing consecutively to prevent COVID-19 but end up in the hospital with an antibiotic-resistant MRSA infection, you've done yourself more harm than good.

» **Don't constantly disinfect your home.** According to the CDC, the general public should routinely clean frequently touched surfaces like doorknobs, handles, light switches, and cellphones to help prevent the spread of the coronavirus. But what does *routinely* entail? I suggest wiping down high-touch surfaces on a daily basis. I don't suggest, however, wiping down these surfaces multiple times a day or scrubbing and disinfecting your entire home on a daily basis (unless someone in your household is already sick). Doing so is unnecessary and may exacerbate any health anxiety you may have.

What's more, most household cleaners are toxic, especially those like bleach that are capable of killing the coronavirus. Continual exposure to chemicals found in household cleaners can irritate lung conditions and may even increase the risk of cancer and birth defects.[24] To stay safe, use cleaning products in well-ventilated areas and wear protective clothing and rubber gloves to protect skin from absorption.

While health anxiety is clearly a serious condition now impacting millions of Americans, no matter how much or little health anxiety you believe you have, worrying too much about your health can make you sick, both physically and mentally. Take the time to identify whether health fears are interfering with your well-being and be proactive about mitigating that anxiety now in our new normal—because the threat of the coronavirus isn't going away. No one should live in fear, and learning to think like a doctor can not only reduce your anxiety but also help you better understand your body and disease pathology so that the world's next pandemic isn't as frightening.

CHAPTER 8

Medical News

At the beginning of the outbreak, as we learned the virus was sickening hundreds in China, Americans began to buy face masks, sometimes in very large quantities. At the time, the CDC, the U.S. surgeon general, and I, along with most other doctors on TV and at patients' bedsides, told Americans we didn't need masks for two reasons: (1) We use masks primarily on sick patients to prevent viral spread to healthy people, so unless you actually have COVID-19, you don't need a mask, and (2) the United States had a severe mask shortage that was already endangering high-risk healthcare workers. No one wanted to see the public, who was at low risk of catching the virus at the time, gut the nation's mask supply like we would eventually decimate store shelves of bleach and toilet paper.

Two months later, however, the CDC flipped its script, announcing that everyone should start to wear face coverings immediately when in public. This abrupt U-turn confused millions, outraged some, and left many feeling betrayed, wondering how

Dr. Anthony Fauci or I could have misled them. I still get angry comments now and then about it on my social media.

So what the heck happened? The answer is something that happens all the time in medicine, but usually doesn't get nearly this much publicity: We learned something new. At the same time, what we already knew didn't change at all. Let me explain. To doctors, new information is known as progress, good science, and good medicine. But given the high profile of the issue and the controversies that have stemmed from it, this reversal in guidance or insight came to be viewed as suspicious, if not incompetent.

After the CDC recommended Americans wear face coverings, I went on ABC to explain why. I told viewers the concept behind the fact that masks were for sick people hadn't changed—that was still a fact. What had changed, however, was that we had learned that up to 45 percent of people infected with COVID-19 show no symptoms, which meant that it was impossible to tell who was sick and who wasn't. In other words, we had to assume that everyone could be sick. There was also still a shortage of surgical masks, which is why the CDC advised people to wear face coverings and not surgical or N95 masks.

The CDC, however, didn't explain that the reversal was based on new information about asymptomatic spread, unfortunately. The same day the CDC announced its new guidelines, President Trump told Americans he would not wear a mask, which raised the volume on the country's confusion.[1] In some ways, I think this personal rejection of CDC recommendations was meant to show that "tough people" don't need to wear masks and that a mask was for the protection of the person wearing it, when the reality was, at that time, the CDC was recommending masks mainly for the protection of others. What's more, false claims—like the CDC originally thought cloth face coverings wouldn't be effective, wearing masks cause oxygen deficiency or can lead to carbon dioxide intoxication, and the agency was really harboring a secret coronavirus cure—circulated like wildfire on the web, further confusing people and complicating the message.

The moral of the mask mix-up is that it's critical to know how to interpret medical news and be able to sort fact from the increasing amount of fiction in our new normal. For decades, Americans have struggled to understand health news and interpret medical headlines. This isn't because they're not intelligent enough or lack the proper education. Instead, medical news is often emotionally threatening, personally impactful, and ever-evolving. That's a lot to unpack in a single article or segment, which can be only 400 words or 20 to 120 seconds long. Additionally, not all doctors, no matter how competent they are in the OR or by the bedside, can effectively communicate information.

In the pandemic era, it's become even more difficult to understand medical news—and a lot easier to fall for fake headlines and false claims. A joint Franklin Templeton–Gallup research project found that many Americans are misinformed, with a "gross misperception of COVID-19 risk"—results that researchers call "stunning" and "shocking."[2] This profound degree of confusion can be detrimental or even deadly.

My job as chief medical correspondent of ABC News is to unpack complex, oftentimes emotionally charged medical news for the public. I've done this on national network TV for fifteen years, but ever since the COVID-19 outbreak began, I've been doing it on a near-daily basis. Because I've been doing it for so long, I can tell you with certainty that the ecosystem around medical news has changed drastically in our new normal, as we've seen an unprecedented uptick in misinformation in health and science. This infodemic has made it more essential to know how to read behind, above, below, around, and through all medical headlines.

Similar to what happens in medicine and science, headlines can suggest something that seems directly contradictory to what we used to think. If we assumed we knew it all in medicine and never reexplored, reanalyzed, or reconsidered our original hypothesis, we would never advance our knowledge base. If we didn't remain open-minded to seeing things differently, learning something new, and changing our recommendations, we would be stuck in the medical and scientific dark ages. The ability to interpret new data or headlines and integrate new information is one character- istic of the scientific mind. Recognizing what is known, as well as what isn't known, is the mark of intellectual integrity. It isn't always about having all the answers; sometimes it's also about ask- ing the right questions. And when you know how to read behind the headlines, you'll be able to better navigate the pandemic era and decipher any important information about your health in the future.

WHEN TOO MUCH INFORMATION BECOMES AN EPIDEMIC

The coronavirus has been malicious in many ways, unseating the world like arguably no other medical, political, or social threat has. But the virus isn't the only enemy we face in our new normal. The amount of misinformation generated by the pandemic has also been devastating, as false claims, unproven treatments, and con- spiracy theories have spread as widely as the virus itself.

At one point, 80 percent of all Americans were exposed to fake news about the virus, according to the Pew Research Center.[3] One team of international researchers discovered more than 2,300 re- ports of rumors, stigma, and conspiracy theories in twenty-five languages and eighty-seven countries, concluding that false claims led to eight hundred deaths and thousands of hospitalizations in the first three months of the outbreak alone.[4]

Today, "we're not just fighting an epidemic; we're fighting an infodemic."[5] That's a quote from the director-general of the

WHO, which recently held a first-ever conference in response to the infodemic. The WHO defines an infodemic as "overabundance of information—some accurate and some not—occurring during an epidemic."[6] No matter what you want to call it, this onslaught of misinformation has deeply troubled the WHO, along with doctors all over the world, including me.

As a physician and the chief medical correspondent of a major national news network, I've been on the front lines in the fight against misinformation with patients and viewers for months. I've been on air almost every day to tell millions of Americans succinctly, accurately, and honestly what I know and don't know about the pandemic.

Never before, however, have I observed so many people asking the same questions, not understanding the news, and feeling confused or even misled by information related to the pandemic. Statistics underscore this observation: While 86 percent of Americans say they follow news about the pandemic "fairly closely," nearly 40 percent say it's become increasingly difficult to know what's true or false about the virus, according to the Pew Research Center.[7]

While some might admit they can't tell fact from fiction when it comes to COVID-19, it hasn't stopped many from trusting inaccurate and potentially harmful claims. In fact, up to 25 percent of all Americans believe fake news about the virus, according to *Scientific American,* and up to 60 percent either identify accurate information as false or can't tell if it's true.[8] Perhaps even more disturbing: One-third of all Americans who've heard the conspiracy theory that the pandemic was planned think it's true, according to the Pew Research Center.[9]

The reasons people don't understand medical information or end up believing misinformation, even material as outrageous as many conspiracy theories for COVID-19, isn't because they're not intelligent. Low health literacy has been a problem for decades, straddling education level, socioeconomic class, political party, and ethnicity. As a doctor, I've seen plenty of highly intelligent patients who simply can't analyze, integrate, or even process medical information.

Many people have a difficult time dealing with medical news because it poses an emotional threat, since the information can affect them both personally and profoundly. In the instance of COVID-19, medical news can literally mean the difference between life and death. That's an immense amount of pressure to get the information right. And when we feel under pressure, intimidated, or scared, it's also often easy to get confused.

These factors—low health literacy and an emotionally charged medical issue—have caused the American public to limp into the pandemic era at a significant disadvantage. Add to this some characteristics unique to COVID-19 and it's easy to see why misinformation has come out swinging in our new normal.

COVID-19 is a new and complicated disease that even doctors have struggled to understand. Even if you strip away COVID-19's complexity, few Americans comprehend the basic principles of infectious disease. The pandemic has forced the public to learn a new lexicon of epidemiological terms like *comorbidities, community transmission,* and *PPE* that were never part of our everyday vocabulary before.

Good data about the disease has also come out at an unprecedented pace, as what we know about the virus has changed on an almost-daily basis. This has caused a degree of informational whiplash. For example, while many were obsessed with disinfecting surfaces at first, after we learned more about how the virus spreads, the CDC stated that fomite transmission—infection through contaminated surfaces—wasn't the primary means of viral spread. This development left many feeling confused and wondering why they had spent weeks smoke-bombing their homes and groceries with disinfectant.

Complex and rapidly evolving data on its own doesn't instigate an infodemic, however. Supply comes on the heels of demand, and in our new normal, we've demanded more medical news than ever before. Whether we want to watch or not, news about the pandemic has become essential: We can't exactly turn a blind eye as to whether there's a mask mandate in our area or a new vaccine that can protect us from serious illness. This makes medical news different from other media buckets like economics, politics, and sports, all of which you can tune out if you're not interested in what the markets are doing, who is lobbying for which legislation, or what team is winning the game.

A problem usually develops, however, whenever demand outstrips supply: All sorts of purveyors magically appear out of the woodwork to fill in the gaps. This has empowered many with a pen or a pulpit to start delivering "news," regardless of whether they have any journalistic cred or medical expertise. Today, so-called experts now interpret complex studies and disseminate medical advice even though they're the chief marketing officer of a tech company or a campaign employee for a political candidate or party. One news outlet even suggests searching "I'm not an epidemiologist, but . . ." on Twitter to see just how many people now espouse medical advice.[10]

Unfortunately, politicians themselves, along with some governmental organizations, have also contributed to the infodemic, spreading disinformation, which is false information or propaganda shared deliberately for personal or political gain. For example, Russian military intelligence has pushed out pandemic propaganda on English-language websites, according to declassified U.S. intelligence,[11] while the European Commission has accused China of spreading disinformation inside the European Union.[12] A handful of American politicians have also made or supported false claims, turning the virus into a political weapon and ratcheting up the country's potential for mistrust.

What's more, not all research, even that which appears in

prominent medical journals, is based on valid science. For example, a commentary published in September 2020 in *The New England Journal of Medicine* suggested that people may be able to immunize themselves against the coronavirus by wearing masks, with the perception that masks expose people to a small amount of the virus at a time almost like a vaccine would.[13] The commentary got a lot of press, but even though *The New England Journal of Medicine* is a very credible publication, the premise of the commentary is simply untrue.

Another example: A Belgian-Dutch team of researchers published a study that subsequently went viral suggesting that runners and cyclists could spread COVID-19 at distances of more than six feet, advocating people stay up to thirty-five feet behind runners and up to sixty-five feet behind those cycling hard.[14] The "study" was self-published and based on computer modeling, not actual research, but it still seeded fear in millions and caused many to stop exercising outdoors.[15] The researchers later admitted that their findings were blown out of proportion.[16]

This is why it matters so much where you get your medical news today—or more specifically, whom you're getting your news from. In the new age of the infodemic, the messenger becomes as important as the message. Because if you can't trust the messenger, you likely can't trust the message, either.

REEVALUATE YOUR MEDICAL NEWS

Whether you already distrust everything you're reading and hearing about the virus—or learning about the infodemic makes you now think twice about medical news—I want you to know that it's important not to give up on medicine or the media. I truly believe that most people in medicine and the established media want to help people, not fool them with fake news or bad science. But you do have to do a little legwork to make sure you're getting your news from a trusted source.

When you see or read medical news, start by asking yourself who, what, where, and how: who's giving the news, what are they saying, where did they get their information, and how was that information determined. You have to put your news under the microscope to understand what you're really consuming and if it's valid.

Focus First on the Who

Of all the who, what, where, and how variables, the most important one when it comes to medical news, in my opinion, is the who: Get the who right and the other factors usually fall into place.

The reason I feel so strongly about the who is that I not only love what I do, I also realize how much is at stake. Whenever I give medical information, it's not just people's health and lives on the line—it's also their trust. When medical news isn't communicated accurately or effectively, people lose faith in medicine or the media altogether. That development, if sustained over the course of someone's lifetime, can be disastrous.

Here are seven steps to help you determine the best "who" to guide you in our new normal:

1. **Ask for credentials.** Credentials establish credibility, which is why you should suss them out immediately in those who deliver medical news. Not everyone is qualified to interpret and present complicated medical information, and degrees of understanding can vary greatly with someone's qualifications. Would you rather get your medical news, for example, from a part-time sports reporter—or a doctor with ten to twenty

years' experience? Similarly, would you rather hear an epidemiologist speak about infectious diseases—or a psychiatrist or veterinarian? Would you rather read a story written by a medical journalist who's written extensively on health and healthcare—or by a junior reporter who also dabbles in entertainment news?

In general, medical doctors tend to have a better understanding of medical information than those who aren't M.D.s. Sometimes people ask me how an OB-GYN can cover medical stories dealing with cancer, COVID-19, or chronic obstructive pulmonary disease (COPD). It's a good question. The answer is simple: In medical school, doctors learn about the entire human body and every specialty. We don't just specialize in one body part or group of body parts—we need to understand the whole body to understand how it connects to that part or group. However, because I am board certified in one specialty, I always—I repeat, *always*—discuss medical stories with colleagues and national experts in the respective fields I cover. Think of it like being an interpreter in a foreign language, that language being Medical.

But not all doctors are competent communicators and can relay information to the public in a way that's understandable, impactful, and empowering. This has nothing to do with a doctor's knowledge base, intelligence level, or clinical experience. You can be the smartest doctor in the room but might not have the knack to communicate emotionally charged information to a lay audience. You can think of it like you do a doctor's bedside manner: Some doctors have it and some don't.

One thing that makes me a successful communicator and helped me achieve the position of chief medical correspondent at a major national network is that I speak *to* viewers—not necessarily at them and never down to them. I speak the same way on the air as I do in my medical practice—in other words, I don't just play a doctor on TV. I have real patients who depend on me, and I speak to them about complex issues in a way that they can digest. Similarly, I always try to make segments relatable and absorbable, and I don't believe in dumbing down the news. I like to tell people what I know and what I don't know so they have all the information to be able to make their own decisions.

2. **Analyze the outlet.** In general, the larger and more prestigious a media outlet, the more scrutiny whoever works for the outlet will face, both externally and internally. I work for ABC News, for example, which is seen by millions of people, including thousands of doctors, agency experts, and researchers. If I got the information wrong, I wouldn't have a job. There's also internal oversight in whatever news I deliver, with a team of medical editors and attorneys fact-checking the material before it goes to air.

3. **Separate actors from part-time players.** Accountability is key. When your job is to appear on air regularly or write frequently for a national publication, you have a reputation to uphold. You need to get it right—this time and every time—or you can lose your job. Established medical journalists who report regularly also know the language to use and don't get sidelined by a camera in front of their faces or the opportunity to have a byline in a major magazine like some part-time players can. Regular correspondents also can't check out whenever they want.

4. **Listen or look for source citations.** Good medical journalists disclose where they get their information, whether it's from a new study, a health organization, or another expert or doctor, or if it's their own professional opinion. On *Good Morning America,* I'll qualify what I say by using phrases like "in my

opinion" or "the CDC recommends." If I spoke with another doctor for insight, I'll identify that person by name and credentials if airtime permits. If my info is based on research, I'll clarify where that study was conducted or published. This way, viewers can assess or determine if the information is legitimate (see more on how to do this on pages 172–75).

5. **Consider the motive.** Medical journalists shouldn't be motivated by personal or professional goals, but it unfortunately can happen—and more so now in the infodemic age. That's why it's so crucial to scrutinize a person's credentials and make sure they deliver the news regularly and qualify their sources—two characteristics that people with an agenda are less likely to do. Also watch out for anyone who speaks in extremes—if something seems too one-sided, it probably is—appears too enthusiastic, or doesn't qualify with simple yet critical words like "may," "can," and "possibly."

6. **Ignore the blowhards.** No one knows everything in medicine and science, and people with professional integrity have no problem admitting that. If someone pretends to know everything or even most things in medicine, you're listening to the wrong messenger. Telling viewers what I know and what I don't know also makes it very clear which areas of information have limitations and may need to be viewed cautiously.

7. **Find someone who doesn't just report, but also explains.** It's one thing to explain the news—it's another to connect the dots to make sure viewers and readers understand how the news might affect them. Look for a journalist who realizes that medical news can be personal and emotional and is able to address you as a person, not as a statistic or an impersonal bystander.

Where *Not* to Get Your Medical News

You now know where to get medical news—or rather, who to get it from. But where shouldn't you turn for trusted medical information? It's quite simple: Stay away from social media, including Facebook, Twitter, YouTube, Instagram, and TikTok. The majority of misinformation spread about the pandemic to date has occurred on these platforms, according to research.[17] Fake posts are also more likely to go viral on social media and be seen, liked, or shared by millions of people.[18]

Facebook, in particular, has proved to be one big hotbed for pandemic misinformation.[19] In August 2020, Facebook revealed it had already removed 7 million posts containing false information about the virus, including some claims about fake preventative treatments and cures.[20] Efforts to stem misinformation haven't been effective, either, with the nonprofit group Avaaz finding 40 percent of coronavirus misinformation remained on Facebook after administrators were alerted that the claims were false.[21]

The bottom line: Don't get your medical news from social media. If you see an interesting article or premise, go to the source or search off social media to learn more. Additionally, think twice before sharing or liking posts about the pandemic, and don't be afraid to contact platform administrators whenever you think a story or account may be spreading misinformation.

Assessing the What, Where, and How

While the messenger matters immensely, it's critical to learn how to evaluate news yourself and be able to spot false claims and inaccurate or exaggerated information. Here are ten questions to ask about any news story to help you assess medical information and uncover the real truth behind the headlines:

1. **Did you really watch or read?** Headlines, anchor introductions, and electronic captions under TV segments are sometimes made to sell the story more than tell the story. That's why it's so important never to take a headline at face value— you have to watch the segment closely or read the entire story. This may sound obvious, but in our ADD era of fast-moving media, few people actually take the time to finish a news story or pay close attention to an entire television segment.

   Case in point: Pew Research Center found that people spend less than one minute reading news articles under 999 words and less than two minutes reading articles between 1,000 and 4,999 words[22]—hardly long enough to comprehend a new or complex topic. If a headline or anchor introduction captivates you, take the time to read it through or listen closely without multitasking. With medical information, the devil is often in the details, and nuances or subtleties can be vitally important.

2. **Is the headline based on new information?** New information is at the core of medicine and science—without it, we'd be stuck diagnosing disease based on outdated criteria, wondering how an infection or illness occurs inside the body, and prescribing drugs or treatments that may not work as well as others. While it can feel unnerving when new information changes the recommended guidance or standard of care, it's

important to realize that this is how good medicine can and does work. Whenever you hear surprising health news where the medical guidance or messaging has changed, ask yourself if it's based on new information or evidence that doctors or researchers didn't know before. If so, pivot and adapt.

3. **Where did the headline originate?** New research often makes medical news, but not all studies are conducted with the same scope and rigor. In general, national health agencies, large hospitals or medical centers, and major academic institutions have the kind of machinery and staff needed to conduct high-quality research. That's why studies conducted at Harvard Medical School or the Cleveland Clinic, for example, tend to carry more weight than research performed by a small college without a medical school, a minor medical center, or a team of doctors with no established affiliation. Keep in mind, too, that almost anyone can conduct a study and hire a publicity team to get the information out to the media, which is why it pays to be discerning about the origins of medical news.

4. **How many outlets are reporting the same headline?** Major networks and publications can get information wrong from time to time. But it's unlikely that multiple major networks or publications will get the same information wrong at the same time in the same way. Compare stories, read or watch closely, and look for subtleties or variations in explanation.

5. **Is the headline a correlation or causation?** *Correlation does not imply causation* and *association is not the equivalent of cause and effect*. Both are Rule No. 1 of statistics and scientific methodology—and why articles claiming that certain foods boost immunity are usually inaccurate (see page 86 for more on this). Here's how it works: When a researcher observes a person has increased immunity after eating an orange, for ex-

ample, that correlation is not the same as the researcher being able to show that oranges improve immunity through X, Y, or Z channel. If this distinction wasn't such a big deal, we might all believe that eating ice cream raises the risk of getting attacked by a shark, since both are more likely to occur on hot, sunny days.

How this understanding can help you in a pandemic is by providing a way to separate facts from unproven possibilities. Let's use the example of so-called COVID toe, or the red, swollen toes doctors began seeing in a small percentage of patients diagnosed with COVID-19. Many people assumed COVID toe was another sign of the disease, but if you applied the correlation-versus-causation test, you'd discover that COVID toe was simply associated with the virus, not necessarily caused by it. As testing for the virus increased in accuracy, researchers discovered that many patients with COVID toe don't actually test positive for the disease, leading them to theorize that red, swollen toes may be a consequence of people wearing shoes less frequently due to more time inside.[23]

6. **Is there a potential conflict of interest?** A lot of newsworthy studies are either conducted or funded by pharmaceutical companies, medical-equipment manufacturers, industry groups, or other businesses with vested interests. This doesn't mean the study is corrupt or invalid, but you should take possible conflicts of interest into account when you consider the conclusions made by the research.

7. **Does the headline sound too good to be true?** When something sounds too good to be true, it often is. For example, many headlines touted homemade cures for COVID-19 at the beginning of the outbreak. While some might sound ridicu-

lous now, that didn't stop plenty of highly intelligent people thinking they could avoid getting the virus by gargling with warm salt water, for example—an early myth made up on social media.[24]

8. **Has the information behind the headline been peer reviewed?** In the new normal, medical information comes out at such a rapid pace that it's not always peer reviewed before it becomes a major headline in the media. Peer-reviewed research means that a team of doctors and scientists have analyzed the study to make sure its methodology and conclusions were well-conducted and logical. You can think of peer-reviewing like *American Idol* for medicine: Experts judge the study and either punch it through to be published, reject it, or ask for revisions, helping to ensure quality control. If the news you're receiving is based on research that hasn't been peer reviewed, that doesn't discount the information, but you should take it with a grain of salt. Also, look for the difference between a study and a commentary. Commentary—as, for example, the piece in *The New England Journal of Medicine* that advocated that masks could be a crude vaccine— means opinion, not science.

9. **What's the sample size?** There's a big difference between exciting news based on a study of thirty thousand people and exciting news concluded from a sample size of thirty. In general, the more patients involved in a clinical study or observational review, the more likely the results are to be accurate. A large sample size lends statistical power to studies and obviates the risk that the results were reached by chance. That's not to say a study conducted on thirty people isn't interesting or worth reporting, but no one should make decisions about their health or standard of care based on such a small sample size.

10. **Does the sample size apply to you?** Here's something that's happened repeatedly in the infodemic age: People draw broad conclusions about a disease based on a study conducted on a unique demographic. In medicine, you can't compare one population with potentially different genetics and life-style factors to another. For example, how the coronavirus impacts people in China may not translate directly to how it affects Americans. Be sure to assess demographic details when you hear or read medical news, and don't automatically draw conclusions between unique populations.

ASSESSING HEADLINES ABOUT NEW DRUGS, DEVICES, AND VACCINES

Few stories have the ability to impact your health like those that detail a new drug, device, or vaccine. Now that we're more than a year into the coronavirus pandemic, we can expect to see more medical news about vaccines and treatments for COVID-19—you can think of it like the next frontier for fake news. It's also the Wild West for bad science, since some researchers—or the countries or corporations that back them—may have something to gain politically or financially by publishing premature or uncorroborated results on new drugs or vaccines. That's why these stories on treatments, devices, and vaccines are often the ones most likely to be sensationalized or include inaccuracies. Here's how to get to the bottom of headlines touting new treatments and try to determine whether a new drug, device, or vaccine might be right for you:

1. **Determine the timeline.** When you hear about a new treatment, the first question to ask is how far away it is from prime time. If someone is extolling a drug that hasn't been tested in humans, you have some time before the treatment will

become available to the public. Make sure the article you're reading or segment you're watching includes information on expected release—if it doesn't, it's probably not a reliable place to get your medical news, as the goal of all responsible medical journalists should be to educate, not instill false hope.

2. **Find out about the follow-up.** The duration of a study can tell you a lot about the hype around a headline. In general, the longer researchers have been studying a drug or device, the better they know and understand its possible outcomes, both favorable and adverse. If researchers or journalists are drawing definitive conclusions about a drug or treatment based on a six-month study, you should have a degree of healthy skepticism.

3. **Make a risks and benefits list.** If you're curious about whether a new drug, device, or vaccine might be right for you, the first step is to speak with a doctor or other qualified healthcare provider. He or she is your best and most reliable source for accurate information.

   While consulting with a doctor, there are also four questions you can ask to help you reach a decision about whether a new drug, treatment, or vaccine might be right for you:

   - What are the risks of doing it?
   - What are the risks of not doing it?
   - What are the benefits of doing it?
   - What are the benefits of not doing it?

In the instance of a COVID-19 vaccine, the risks of vaccination might include experiencing mild side effects. The risks of not getting vaccinated might include possible infection, serious illness, and/or death from the disease, as well as possible transmission to others. The benefits of vaccination might include reduced possibility of infection, serious illness, death, and transmission, along with potential peace of mind and the ability to participate in public or social activities that require vaccination. The benefits of not getting vaccinated might include experiencing no vaccine-related side effects. A risk-benefits analysis can usually help to clarify confusion or distill the noise around potentially controversial medical decisions.

A pandemic by nature is an incredibly challenging time. If you don't understand the information or can't find reliable sources for your medical news, the consequences can be grave. On the other hand, learning to find trusted sources and interpret medical headlines can help you navigate more smartly and safely through our new normal. These skills will also make it easier for you to interface with doctors and understand medical concerns you may face in the future. Think of it like learning a few words in another language before you travel through a foreign country: Our new normal is foreign to us all, and the sooner we can adjust to the landscape, the easier it will be for us to adapt and thrive.

CHAPTER 9

Family and Friends

In pre-pandemic times, we interacted with friends and family how, when, and where we wanted. Today, in our new normal, our friends are all possible pathogen threats and family falls into two groups: Those we worry we might make sick, like our parents, grandparents, and newborn babies, and everyone else, whom we fear we might get sick from.

Never before have we had to scrutinize our closest relationships so carefully, evaluating the health behaviors and risk tolerance of others in order to make tough decisions about whom we will and won't see. In the B.C. (before coronavirus) years, we had friend groups and extended family. Now we have pandemic pods—small, self-contained circles of people with whom we socialize exclusively. We judge others based on whether they wear a mask, and we worry about sharing a bed with a spouse or romantic partner who goes into an office or out to a crowded bar. We agonize over whether to see our elderly parents and fret about allowing our children to go to a playground or birthday party. We even worry whether our dogs and cats might get sick—or make us sick.

This is an entirely new way of thinking. Most of us have never had to assess our health and daily behaviors relative to the health and daily behaviors of every person we meet. This happened to some degree at the height of the HIV epidemic, when every sexual partner posed a possible danger and it was imperative to take precautions, ultimately trusting the person you were with.

Today, we're taking similar safeguards, but the threat is no longer just sharing the same bed, it's sharing the same breathing space as well. Everyone has become patient zero, as we look sideways at family and friends, wondering where they've been, whom they've been with, and whether they've been safe. It sounds a lot like STDs, except the fallout and emotional anxiety, judgment, and stigma is all-inclusive this time.

Of course, there is concern, too. Many have had to put the health of others in front of their own convenience or needs. That's a beautiful thing to behold in our new normal, even if it's required some painful sacrifices at times.

I'm in a unique position as a doctor, but I still make challenging decisions every day about how to interact with family and friends. My parents, for example, are eighty, healthy, and part of a small pod. They aren't seeing a lot of people, which is a major adjustment for them, but they still see me—and I go into my office, see patients, and am always in the ABC News studio. When I get together with my parents, I mandate that we eat outside as much as possible, weather permitting. We wear masks and remain at least six feet apart, which takes a lot of effort on my end.

Despite the fact that both my parents are retired medical professionals, I have to remind them to keep their distance and not pull down their masks while talking. My mother also rolls up the windows when I drive her, even though I insist on keeping them down to improve ventilation and protect her. She tells me she doesn't want to live like this and that if she gets sick, she gets sick. But I certainly don't want her to get sick, and neither do my children, Alex and Chloe.

Managing risks with Alex and Chloe has been easier than for some parents of college-age kids. I'm fortunate that my kids understand what's at stake in a pandemic and are responsible about their behaviors. What helped is that we all agreed at the beginning of the outbreak that their significant others would be part of our family pod. Today, I don't worry about them because I know they're not going out to bars or parties or taking other unnecessary risks. They wear masks, stay at least six feet apart, and don't go to crowded, public places.

None of this is to say their lives have been easy in the new normal. Chloe opted out of her sophomore year at Harvard University after the school canceled in-person classes and the Ivy League canceled fall sports—an important aspect of her college career, since she plays for the Crimson ice hockey team. And both Chloe and Alex have had to make tough decisions about their social lives that I wouldn't have thought would be the new norm for young people. One of my children, for example, agonized for days over whether to see a group of friends who clearly weren't taking the pandemic seriously. In the end, my kid chose not to get together with these close friends. I was floored: These were college kids saying no to things like meeting for pizza or taking a hike outside, not because of drugs, sex, or alcohol, but because of potential viral exposure. That's what our new reality looks like, and it's been very hard.

Being the parent of young kids poses a whole other set of problems in pandemic times. In the instance of COVID-19, while many parents (and even some public health officials) mistakenly assumed they didn't have to worry extensively about young children, we now know better: Kids can and do get infected and transmit the virus to adults, other children, and other families, creating a potentially far-reaching ripple effect of viral spread. This has caused many to fret over what children, who have a hard time practicing safety precautions, should be allowed to do, creating fissures between families, school administrators, and communities at large.

These fissures have led to social stigma, judgment, and even ostracization, all of which are acute issues in our new normal. I see it every day in my friend circle. Recently, for example, a friend posted a photo on social media of two cousins sharing a chair without masks, which they'd taken off only for the photo. But after one of the girls' mother saw the picture, she demanded her daughter be tested immediately (this defies the viral principle of a latency period, or the time between exposure and infection) and now won't allow her to see her cousin. Another friend who is an ER doc with ten-year-old twins can find only one other family in her friend group willing to let their children play together—other parents say they're too worried about her exposure, even though most doctors know how to manage their health risks much better than the general public.

The pandemic is also changing marital and romantic relationships, driving a wedge between some couples while bringing others closer together. I'm lucky to have a boyfriend who is an infectious disease doc: We share the same risk tolerance, and he certainly knows how to stay safe in a contagious outbreak. At the same time, since we don't live together, we've had to overcome the challenge of navigating a new exposure every time we meet. During the initial outbreak, we agreed to get tested for COVID-19 whenever we saw each other, but this quickly became unsustainable (we did it once), and we've since learned how to stay safe together, learning how to use surveillance testing more strategically as our exposures increased. Married couples and those who do live together naturally have different concerns, including what to do when one gets sick and you have no other choice but to share the same bed.

To me, managing all these relationships feels a little like having to draw a Venn diagram over and over again, widening or reducing the area of overlap where the circles of ourselves, family members, and friends all intersect. Some people want a very small area of overlap; others are clearly comfortable with a much wider circle of intersection. But only you know how big you want your over-lapping area to be in your pandemic diagram. Neither Dr. Anthony Fauci nor your family physician nor I can tell you who to let into your life and by how much. Instead, these decisions should be based partly on your health and the health of those around you, but also on your risk tolerance and what or whom you believe to be worth taking a chance for in our new normal.

Still, as an expert in medical science risk management, I can help guide you to make smarter decisions about who, how, and when to spend time with others. In this chapter, you'll learn how to manage and mitigate risks with older relatives, marital or romantic partners, friends, pets, and children of all age groups, including newborns, young kids, preteens, and teenagers and college-age students. While no one can give you a numerical percentage of what your actual risk is of seeing X person or Y individual, I can help you understand how to stratify your risk and weigh the factors involved in various social encounters. The goal of this chapter isn't to help you select your pandemic pod, but to show you how to stay happy, healthy, and connected in a new world where we'll have to think twice about how we socialize for years to come.

EIGHT RULES FOR SOCIALIZING IN OUR NEW NORMAL

No matter your risk tolerance or whom you want to spend time with, there are a few ground rules to consider when socializing with others in our new normal. Getting together with family and friends is emotionally loaded and will be for months to come, even after certain guidelines are relaxed. Some people will always remain fearful, others may become more dismissive, and many will float somewhere in between, but there's no way to predict someone else's risk tolerance and when or if it might change. This makes basic etiquette key to both healthy and happy social interactions. Some of the following eight rules can help you stay safe, while others may help you retain certain relationships without angering or offending others.

1. **Recognize there's always a risk.** Unless you spend the rest of your life inside a sterile bubble, you can never bring your risk level down to zero, even if everyone gets tested (false negatives) and vaccinated (no vaccine is 100 percent). There will always be the chance of someone getting infected with COVID-19 or any other contagious illness, including coughs and colds, the flu, strep throat, stomach viruses, measles, whooping cough, and dozens of other diseases. What you can do, however, is control the controllables, which means doing everything you can realistically and sustainably to lower your risk level to as low as possible.

2. **Don't do it if you're sick.** This should be obvious by now, but we all know that person who comes to Thanksgiving with a cough or shows up in the office or at a birthday party only hours after recovering from a stomach flu. This behavior wasn't cool before COVID-19, and it's just downright dangerous now. Bottom line: Stay home if you feel sick. If you suspect you may have COVID-19 or another contagious illness, call your doctor and wait at least one to two weeks before seeing other people.

3. **Ask before you assume.** Don't think that just because a friend or relative is ostensibly healthy that he or she will be okay if you go in for a hug or come closer than six feet. Ask those around you before having any unmasked, close, or direct contact. If they don't want to interact, don't be offended. Recognize that someone's individual health, risk factors for

COVID-19, and unique risk tolerance are deeply personal and have nothing to do with you and/or how much they may want to see you.

4. **Mask up when not with your pod.** Always wear a mask and keep your distance when you're with anyone who's not in your pandemic pod, in addition to people over age sixty-five, newborns, and those with compromised immune systems. Remember that it's not one or the other: The CDC recommends wearing masks and staying at least six feet apart to help prevent the spread of this infectious respiratory disease.

5. **Get out.** Anything you can do outside or in a well-ventilated area will be safer than activities done inside, especially in poorly ventilated rooms. Remember that you're trying to stop the spread not only of COVID-19, but of many other infectious illnesses, too.

6. **Stop with the chips and dip.** It's human nature to want to share food and drinks at get-togethers with family and friends. But in our new normal, communal snacks that people eat with their hands like chips and dip, popcorn, and nuts should be off-limits. In addition, don't share plates, silverware, or glasses, and remain aware when splitting appetizers or meals with others at restaurants.

7. **Talk boundaries beforehand.** Getting together in our new normal can be tense, awkward, and uncomfortable. People are sensitive and will be for a while. The best way to avoid offending friends and family or potentially alienating relationships important to you is to talk before you visit in order to discuss their boundaries and yours when it comes to COVID-19. If you don't know the person well enough to have a conversation before you see them, be respectful when you visit by keeping your mask on and staying at least six feet apart.

8. **Make it about you, not them.** If you don't feel comfortable seeing someone in person, politely explain your feelings, emphasizing that you're making the decision to protect *your* health. Even if you believe the other person is taking unnecessary risks, you don't need to share that with them to decline an invite. If you make it about you and your health, the other person is less likely to feel judged or offended. If you refuse an in-person invite, suggest an alternative. If you don't feel comfortable attending a dinner party, for example, offer to call in via video to say hello to the guests before everyone sits down to eat. Or if you don't want to attend a wedding, communicate with the couple that you'd love to see photos or the wedding video once available.

SPENDING TIME WITH PEOPLE OVER AGE SIXTY-FIVE

The relationships that seem to be causing the most anxiety in our new normal are the ones we have with our older relatives and friends. The concern is valid: Age is the single biggest risk factor for serious complications from COVID-19, and eight out of every ten COVID-19 deaths in the United States to date have occurred in people age sixty-five years or older.[1] Older people are also much more susceptible to the flu and other infectious illnesses.

If you're going to spend time with older family members or friends, you should be cautious about if, when, how, and where you'll do so. Here are my guidelines to help you make the decision and safely see older people if you decide it's sensible to do so.

Make the Decision

Visiting an older relative or friend in our new normal is a decision to make, not a privilege to take. The first step is to speak with the older relative or friend and determine if he or she feels comfortable with an in-person visit. If the person doesn't feel safe, don't feel hurt or angry or try to pressure them. Remember that everyone has a different risk tolerance and the right to be protective of their health and well-being.

If an older relative or friend is comfortable with your visit, you should still weigh the risks of whether doing so is actually prudent in our new normal. Here are three variables to consider in making your decision:

» **Their risk factors:** The older they are, the bigger their risk of infectious illness in general. The chance of dying from COVID-19, for example, increases drastically with each decade: Those who are eighty-five and older have a 630 times higher chance of death from the disease, while those in the sixty-five to seventy-four age bracket have only a 90 times higher chance.[2] Similarly, older people who are overweight or obese or suffer from heart disease, diabetes, high blood pressure, or another health ailment are much more vulnerable to getting seriously sick.

» **Your exposure:** We all have varying degrees of exposure to infectious illness. A person who lives with a big family, works outside the home, and/or doesn't wear a mask has a greater chance of contracting a bacterial infection or virus than a person who lives alone, works from home, and/or always takes precautions. Consider your daily activities as well: Going to gyms, restaurants, bars, and other indoor places boosts your chance of exposure to illness. Similarly, if you live in a COVID-19 hot spot and are traveling to see an older relative or friend in an area with a relatively low case rate, your exposure will be comparatively much greater.

» **The visit:** How and where you visit can significantly increase or decrease the risk level. For example, do you plan to visit for two hours or two weeks? Can you see the older person only outside or will you need to be indoors, too? Will you be in a house where everyone can stay at least six feet apart, or does your older relative or friend live inside a small apartment? In the instance of COVID-19, can you isolate for up to two weeks or get tested before you go?

If you weigh your conclusions from these three variables, you should be able to reach a decision fairly confidently about whether to visit an older friend or relative. Remember that you'll never be able to obviate the risk entirely, but you can take every step possible to mitigate the likelihood of disease transmission by asking everyone to wear a mask when visiting or getting testing before you go.

Treat Them Like a Newborn Baby

If you've ever visited a newborn baby, you likely know that you can't just smother them with kisses and put your hands all over them. Think of older family and friends in the same way and avoid kissing, hugging, and other forms of direct contact.

It's Okay to Say You're Worried

While you might be anxious about getting an older person sick, they may not share your concern. Many baby boomers and elderly adults in our new normal aren't taking their health seriously, refusing to wear a mask and continuing to socialize like it's 2019. Some feel as though they've seen it all and are invulnerable to disease, while others would rather chance getting sick than give up their autonomy or way or life. Either way, the obstinacy has left millions of younger people fearful for their safety.

If you're worried about an older relative or friend, talk to them rationally and reasonably about your concerns. Use facts, not fear tactics, to explain why you'd like them to take certain precautions, and ask how you can make it easier or more sustainable for them.

If they're unwilling to be safe for their own sake, ask them to do it for you and others who want to enjoy their company for years to come.

Why Nursing Homes Are Different

Older people who live in nursing homes have one of the highest death rates of COVID-19, not just because of their age, but also due to the fact that the facilities are often revolving doors between staff, visitors, and residents coming from hospitals and homes. If you want to visit a relative or friend in a nursing home, I suggest you carefully consider your exposure and the risk-benefit ratio. If you decide to go, call ahead to find out if the facility is mandating any special precautions. Upon arrival, be prepared to have your temperature checked and/or to fill out a surveillance questionnaire. Once inside, always wear your mask, keep at least six feet away whenever possible, and wash your hands frequently and meticulously. Be aware, too, that masks and limitations on visitors may be permanent precautionary measures for many homes.

STAYING SAFE WITH CHILDREN

There's a saying in pediatrics I learned in medical school that I've repeated often on air during the pandemic: Kids aren't little adults. That's why the specialty of pediatrics exists. You can't just take adult diseases, shrink them down to fit inside a smaller body, and expect the results to be the same. The coronavirus is a perfect example of this.

Here's why: After early reports found children weren't get-

ting seriously sick with COVID-19, many parents and some doctors misinterpreted the headlines to mean kids don't get the virus,
which isn't true (another example of why it's important to read
behind headlines—see chapter 8 to learn how). Both Dr. Fauci
and I, among others, tried to correct the misperception on TV,
telling viewers that children can and do get infected, but most
don't become as seriously ill or have anywhere near the same
death rate as do adults with the disease, though there are deaths
among children. But the damage had already been done, priming
the pump for some future missteps surrounding kids in our new
normal.

While we're still figuring out the role children play in viral
transmission, we now know that kids can and do get COVID-19,
and just like adults, spread the disease to others. Children also
appear more likely to have mild symptoms or be asymptomatic,
making it more likely that they'll be silent spreaders of the virus.
Kids may also have higher viral loads than adults[3] and shed the
virus for weeks after becoming infected, which may or may not
increase their ability to transmit the disease.[4] Moreover, kids never
live alone: They live with parents, grandparents, and/or other care-
takers who can, do, and have become seriously ill with COVID-19.

Even within the specialty of pediatrics, it's not one size fits all.
There are extraordinary physical, mental, and emotional differences between toddlers and teens, and all age groups have different
distinct risk factors when it comes to COVID-19. These variables
should influence how you interact with children, whether you're
a parent, relative, or friend. Here, we'll address four different
age groups—newborns and infants, children under age ten, preteens, and high school and college-age kids—and tell you what
you need to know to keep each group safe in our new normal. I
will take you through the aspects that make COVID-19 in pediatric age groups unique, distinctive, and emotionally charged. In
understanding the subtle and developmental differences between

different age groups, you can better navigate these challenging and ever-evolving issues.

Newborns and Infants

Babies rely on their mothers for a substantial part of their immune system. They receive antibodies in utero and via breast milk, along with some protection from vaccinations. But their immune systems are still very immature, and if they get sick with anything, the outcome can be far more severe than if an older child contracts the same illness.

For this reason, you should be very careful around newborns and infants in our new normal, just as you should have been before the pandemic. If you're a parent, limit or avoid visitors altogether for at least the first month after your child's birth. You'll also want to keep your pandemic pod very small to reduce your overlapping area of exposure. If you have any reason to suspect you may have COVID-19, the flu, or any other contagious illness, speak with your obstetrician or pediatrician and be prepared to temporarily separate or distance yourself from your baby—the risk of giving your child an infectious disease likely outweighs the risk of not participating in parental bonding.

If you'd like to visit a newborn, talk with the baby's parents beforehand to make sure they're comfortable with the encounter. Be sure that you're healthy and asymptomatic for at least one week before you see the baby. While you don't have to change into a sterile hospital gown when you go, wear a mask and wash your hands frequently and thoroughly. You'll also want to minimize close contact with the child, as well as his or her parents, who can spread whatever you give them to their baby. If you're close family, it may be okay to hold an infant for a few minutes. But if you're not close family, I'd ask yourself if it's really necessary for you to hold the baby, even if the parents are amenable. Either way, don't kiss a newborn, especially on his or her face or hands, which will go straight inside the child's mouth.

What to Do If You're Pregnant During a Pandemic

Most women are likely taking a number of precautions already to protect their health and well-being if they're expecting. But during a pandemic, you may need to be even more cautious about what you do, where you go, and whom you see. Because pregnant women are considered to have a compromised or suppressed immune system, they're more susceptible to infections, which may include COVID-19. Keep in mind that you're not the only patient, but that your fetus's well-being could be compromised if you become seriously ill while pregnant. Even if you're young and healthy, err on the side of safety. If you have specific concerns, talk to your obstetrician and/or midwife—good communication will help ensure everything goes as smoothly as possible during both your pregnancy and delivery.

Children Ages One to Nine

At baseline, young children are difficult to control. They don't follow directions well, their overall hygiene isn't great, they constantly touch their faces and everything around them, they don't understand personal space, and they need to be supervised in nearly everything they do. Young children also don't have well-developed fine motor skills, which can lead to difficulties when washing hands, putting on a mask, and trying not to touch handles, railings, adults, and other possible supporting objects.

Despite these realities, it's still very important that kids wear masks, wash their hands well, and practice social distancing. Young children can get COVID-19, and even while they don't usually get seriously sick and the fatality rate is very, very low, they can still pass the disease on to parents, grandparents, and other possibly vulnerable adults. Young children also appear less likely than older kids to show symptoms of COVID-19, increasing the likelihood they'll be silent spreaders.

What's more, children in this age range are more likely to have close contact with other kids, which can immediately and dramatically widen your circle of risk if they're not social distancing and wearing masks. Keep in mind, too, that some children may have preexisting medical conditions, making them more vulnerable to severe complications with COVID-19. Finally, young children can develop multisystem inflammatory syndrome, a rare but serious condition associated with COVID-19.[5]

I realize that teaching and enforcing safety precautions in this age group can be a tall order. But I believe that if kids can be taught how to use a toilet, they can learn how to wear a mask and keep their distance from others. It's not easy, but neither is toilet training. And similar to toilet training, once young children learn how to do it, they can usually adhere without continual oversight.

Whether you teach your kids safety precautions may play a role in the bigger decisions so many parents face in our new normal: Is it okay to let children engage in the group activities that are so important for their development, including in-person classes, day care, team sports, music or dance lessons, summer camp, and similar events with other children and adults?

To help make this decision, I suggest you look within and without. What do I mean? Looking within means assessing the health of everyone in your pandemic pod. Is everyone generally healthy?

Does anyone have any preexisting conditions, including obesity, that would put them at a higher risk of severe complications with COVID-19? Are grandparents or older relatives helping to care for your child? Do you regularly visit older adults?

Next, look without, which means evaluating the risk of activities in your community. What is the infection rate of COVID-19 or other contagious illnesses in your area? Is the activity being held outside, inside, or in a well-ventilated space? Will everyone be wearing masks? Will teachers or supervising adults help keep kids apart or at least discourage hugging and other close contact?

Now, consider the worst-case scenario: your child gets infected and exposes your pandemic pod. If your pandemic pod is relatively healthy and/or low risk, the activity is low risk, and/or there's not a lot of infectious illness in your area, it may be okay to have your child participate in group activities.

What about individual playdates during a pandemic? This has been a loaded question for many parents in our new normal, with families sizing one another up and often making uncomfortable judgments about each other's health behaviors and practices. This in turn has led to many disagreements, social stigma, and ostracism.

From a medical perspective, I would advise you to find families who share your health practices and level of risk tolerance. It's okay to ask questions. In our new normal, no one should be offended if you want to know whether everyone wears masks when out in public or has been vaccinated.

Whether it's playdates or group activities, keep in mind that you'll never be able to bring the risk down to zero. What's more, there are significant mental, emotional, and even physical detriments to keeping kids out of school or away from other children. Finally, remember that there are risks in everything your child does. You can choose to keep your kid home out of fear of COVID-19, but then he or she might have a bad fall, get burned,

or accidentally ingest something poisonous, all of which are leading causes of injury in this age group.[6]

Children Ages Ten to Fourteen

The same safety measures for younger children also apply to this
age group: Everyone should be wearing masks, washing their
hands frequently, and physically distancing. Preteens can be infected with COVID-19 and don't often show symptoms, so they
can also transmit the virus unknowingly to adults and other kids.

Unlike younger children, however, this age bracket is more
mature and will usually listen to direction. They are also more
likely to be able to fully comprehend why it's necessary to wear
a mask, for example, if it's explained to them. At the same time,
many preteens are very impressionable, so they're more apt to follow guidance than older teens. In a way, this makes this age group
the "sweet spot" for adopting safety measures in a pandemic.

To take advantage of these attributes, parents should (1) explain the facts, and (2) be specific about which measures they want
their preteens to take. Have a mature conversation with your kids,
telling them what we know about the virus (or any another illness)
and how they can transmit the illness without knowing it. Be clear
that they can spread the disease without feeling sick, which could
make other people very sick. Focus on facts, not fear, and ask them
to share their feelings and concerns in our new normal.

High School and College-Age Kids

With teens and young adults, it's critical to know your patient
population. Otherwise, if you treat this age group like you would
younger kids or older adults, you'll miss the mark 99 percent of
time. Whether you're a parent, relative, or friend of the family,
leveraging the psychology of high school and college-age kids can

help you better guide their behavior and keep everyone healthier and happier in our new normal.

As you likely know, the teenage years are when children exert their independence, separate from their parents, and question or even challenge authority. They may struggle to find their identity, learn how to manage their emotions, and develop more mature relationships outside the family.

Parenting teens and young adults was challenging in pre-pandemic times, but in our new normal, managing this age group can be particularly tough. The last thing any teenager wants is to be told what to do. Their social lives are their lifeblood, and they want to see their friends. As they try to establish their identity, many don't want to wear a mask that makes them look like everyone else. They long for close contact and many want to start exploring their sexuality, too. All of this is normal behavior.

My advice for this age group is what good doctors do with all patients: start with honest and open communication. Recognize that while the pandemic is difficult on everyone, it's especially tough for them, socially and developmentally. I believe you have to acknowledge this—otherwise, they may not hear anything else you say.

As you would with preteens, explain the science behind the disease and what we know about this age group's role in transmission, or that they can spread the disease easily and unknowingly to you, the rest of your family, their teachers, their friends, and their friends' families. Since this age group can be self-absorbed, take the time to emphasize that being safe isn't about them—it's about everyone around them and the greater good. Tell them that this is their time to step up and prove they can be adults in a situation that requires both maturity and responsibility. After all, part of being an adult means doing what we need and should do, even if it isn't what we want to do.

When you talk with teens or young adults, be direct about the specific precautions you want them to take. At the same time, be realistic about your expectations: Know that you likely can't control everything they do. Ask them to stay at least six feet apart from their friends, but emphasize that seven feet is better than six feet, and both are better than six inches. If they're resistant to wearing a mask, encourage them to find a face covering that lets them express their personality, either by color, fashion, or design.

You can also ask your teen or college-age kid what you can do to make the pandemic more sustainable for them. For example, I agreed to include my kids' significant others in our pandemic pod, which made it immensely easier on all of us. (This was possible since technically my "kids" aren't really kids: They are twenty-two and twenty-one, but of course they will always be kids to me.) You might also consider offering a diversion within your home or family that could help compensate for the activities they can't do. For example, adopting a dog or cat and making the pet your teen's responsibility may make it easier for him or her to stay home. Similarly, maybe there's a project your kid could do, like repainting his or her room or caring for younger children in exchange for a small fee.

Finally, keep in mind that many teens and young adults are anxious or scared in our new normal, even if they don't show it. Half my patients are under age twenty-one, and many have broken down in the exam room, admitting to feeling stressed and anxious since the world as they knew it has been turned upside down. Be sensitive to how your child might feel and encourage them to talk about their emotions, whether it's with you or a trained therapist.

What to Do If You Test Positive

If you test positive for COVID-19, the first thing to do is go home and isolate yourself. The second thing to do is pick up the phone and call everyone you've had any close contact with in the last forty-eight hours, including those at work and/or establishments like restaurants, gyms, churches, or salons. While making these calls may not be easy, it's absolutely necessary—and ultimately much easier than living with the fear you may have allowed a friend or relative to spread the disease to dozens of others. If you feel guilty, embarrassed, or scared, it's okay to be honest and admit on the phone how you're feeling. You may be surprised that your friends and family are more understanding than you think.

NAVIGATING MARRIED OR ROMANTIC RELATIONSHIPS

The pandemic has injected many marriages and other romantic relationships with stress, social isolation, financial uncertainty, parental difficulties, and/or intimacy issues, all of which are here to stay for the long haul. The upshot has been mixed, deepening some relationships while causing others to break apart. Unmarried couples seem to be weathering the storm better than married folk, with seven of out ten unmarried people reporting that their relationship has become more serious since the outbreak began, according to a survey from Ipsos.[7]

These couples, however, may be the exception, not the norm. Anecdotal evidence from divorce attorneys shows a surge of interest in marital separation[8] while the same Ipsos survey found that one in ten married or partnered unions in the United States are very likely to separate due to issues related to the pandemic.[9] One in five couples are also now fighting more while 27 percent of all Americans say they know a couple who is likely to break up, separate, or divorce whenever the pandemic ends.[10]

As I've said many times on *Good Morning America,* crises tend to bring out the best and worst in people, and it's often our significant others who are the first to see these extremes. Navigating interpersonal problems hasn't been and never will be easy, especially if one or both people in a relationship are experiencing any of the mental-health issues common in our new normal. My best advice is to communicate, communicate, communicate. Tell your partner how you're feeling, whether that's scared, stressed, or suffocated, without blaming the other person. Explain your needs with empathy and compassion for your spouse or partner, who's also been through a stressful time, and ask what he or she may need right now to feel healthy and happy.

No matter your situation with your spouse or partner, don't let health concerns add to your anxiety or problems. If you or your partner gets sick, don't share the same bed. This was good advice before COVID-19, but it's become even more critical since sleeping in same bed for up to eight hours at a time is one of the most intense forms of close contact you can have with someone else. When someone in a relationship gets sick, concede the bedroom to the person who isn't feeling well—the healthy partner can spend the night in a spare bedroom or on the couch. Don't be intimate while sick and for up to approximately ten days after the first sign of symptoms.

Sex and the Single Person in Pandemic Times

Can I date during a pandemic? Can I have sex during a pandemic? These are the questions I hear on a regular basis from almost every one of my single patients. My answer: There is no easy answer. It's a tricky and sticky situation, and there's always a risk in everything you do. But you can use good judgment to lower your risk. You can think of it with almost the same decision-making criteria you would use to reduce your chance of getting a sexually transmitted infection.

Start by being selective about whom you date. Do they share the same health behaviors and risk tolerance as you do? You probably don't want to date someone who doesn't believe in masks if you do, for example, or has no problem going out to crowded bars all night while you're social distancing. Also ask yourself how important the relationship is to you. While it's probably worth the risk to see someone you really like and foresee a future with, it might not be smart to take the same chances on a guy or gal who may be in your life for only a few weeks.

SPENDING TIME WITH FRIENDS

A pandemic is a socially charged situation for all our relationships: When someone else can give you a potentially debilitating disease, every acquaintance gets reassessed. But pandemics may exact a particular toll for friends, who are people we want to see but may not necessarily need to see, which has forced many to reevaluate their friendships six ways to Sunday. For this reason, many friendships have fallen apart in our new normal, as people disagree over risk tolerances and health behaviors or simply don't see each other anymore. Conversely, the crisis has also deepened some friendships, as people have come together in a shared time of need.

I'm a medical doctor, not a therapist, so I can't tell you how to heal your friendships. But I can give you etiquette to follow when it comes to navigating the health behaviors of your friends. Here are seven tips to keep in mind when you spend time with people outside your pandemic pod:

1. **Opt at times for a party of one.** We shouldn't have to keep saying it, but we will: stay home if you're sick. While some may apply a different filter for when they want to socialize with friends, sharing is not caring in the age of contagious disease.

2. **Huddle before you hang.** When meeting with a friend or group of friends, intentionally start a conversation about which safety precautions will make everyone feel comfortable. This way, you know how your friends feel and can avoid missteps that might offend someone or make another feel uncomfortable. Talking also allows you to communicate how you feel so that your friends can respect your safety measures.

3. **Accept the highest common denominator.** If a friend has a particular safety concern—e.g., they don't want to go to a restaurant, they don't feel comfortable inside—respect that concern and adhere to their wishes whenever together. Think of it like wearing a seat belt in someone else's car or taking your shoes off when you go inside a friend's home: If that's what they want you to do, the polite thing to do is to nod, smile, and comply.

4. **Respect the RT.** Everyone has a unique risk tolerance, which was true before the pandemic began. For example, you may have a friend who would happily sky dive out of a plane as well as one who wouldn't even get inside a small plane, let alone jump out of one. Respect your friends' personal boundaries.

5. **Don't assume motives.** Sometimes a friend may want to take measures you feel are excessive not to protect themselves, but to protect a vulnerable family member or friend. You may never know their motives unless you walk in their shoes, but the thing to do is not get upset or hurt by what they feel they need to do.

6. **More is better.** When in doubt, err on the side of safety. In our new normal, no one is going to accuse you of being rude if

you want to stay at least six feet apart. Similarly, you'll never be sorry if everyone wears a mask inside a restaurant, but you may be if someone gets sick if you didn't.

7. **You can choose you.** It's okay to prioritize your health over a friendship, especially if someone is unwilling to respect your boundaries. If that's the case, they're likely not a true friend anyway.

Playing It Safe with Furry Friends

Sometimes there's no greater relationship than the one we have with man's (and woman's) best friend: our pets. First, the bad news: COVID-19 can infect dogs and cats. Since it's a coronavirus, we know that some strains affect animals. But confirmed cases are rare, and reported deaths from the disease are even more unusual. Most pets don't show symptoms, or if they do, they're very mild. What's more, the risk of your pet spreading the illness to you is low, according to the CDC.[11] The risk is likely greater that you could spread the virus to your pet. While it's possible to test your dog or cat for COVID-19, the CDC recommends doing so only if your pet exhibits symptoms associated with the virus and has had known contact with an infected individual.[12] If you're sick with COVID-19 or any other illness, avoid sleeping in the same bed or kissing or hugging your pet.

In the end, one of the biggest changes wrought by the pandemic is how to interact with other people. Our new normal has transformed our relationships with family and friends, and it's not easy to know who to see and how to socialize. But you don't have to be reactive about relationships in our new normal. Instead, you can choose to make conscious, informed, and smart decisions about who you see and how you see them. Doing so will greatly increase the chances that you and your family will stay safe while staying connected with the people who matter most in your new world.

CHAPTER 10

Public Places

Captain Dennis Tajer flies several days every week. He does it because he has to—it's his job as a 737 pilot—but he also does it because he wants to. In our new normal, Tajer says he's confident that his profession doesn't put his health at risk.

"It's ironic that people will go to restaurants where the airflow is standard, and they'll feel comfortable taking down their masks and eating. But they think twice about being on an airplane, where airflow goes through a HEPA filter and is superior," Tajer recently told me by phone. "Everyone should feel safe on a plane. That's engineering—that's not opinion."

I saw Tajer—at least on TVs at the station—when we featured him on *Nightline* in May 2020. ABC News transportation correspondent Gio Benitez caught up with Tajer then, the day the pilot started flying after being grounded for weeks due to the COVID-19 outbreak. Months after the segment aired, Tajer told me those early weeks had been a struggle, before the airlines implemented widespread mask mandates. But today, the spokesman for the union group the Allied Pilots Association says everyone he sees on a plane and in an airport is wearing a mask over their nose and mouth—a game changer for air-travel safety in our new normal.

"I couldn't engage in this on a day-to-day basis if I felt my passengers were unsafe—not just morally, but professionally, I couldn't fly a plane," Tajer said. "I make that obligation every time I clip on those wings."

There's wisdom behind these words—Tajer has been flying passenger planes for more than thirty years. In those three decades, he's never seen anything affect air travel like the pandemic—and he says the outbreak will keep shaping the air-travel industry for years to come.

"You can't go through this and not have it change your life," he told me. "It's part of the human experience. There's going to be a period of time when people feel more comfortable wearing a mask, whether it's COVID-19 or not. I think people are going to take these precautions out of personal choice."

In the meantime, Tajer says no one should feel afraid to fly in our new normal. But if you're hesitant, he says he understands. "It's okay to feel that way," he told me. "It takes time, and everyone is going to have a process to get to the point where they feel comfortable. But when you're ready, we'll be ready for you."

Tajer is right: There's a process and it does take time. Answering the question of whether it's safe to fly—or go back to work, the gym, a restaurant, a theater, a salon, a church, or any other public place—starts with one variable: you. Because only you can make the decision.

But there are specific ways to assess your risk and evaluate the safety of any situation for yourself and/or loved ones. In this chapter, we'll look at four factors to consider whenever you go to crowded public places and distinct ways to protect yourself in our new normal, whether you're headed back to work, taking a trip, eating at a restaurant, going to a salon, attending a religious service, or enjoying a museum, movie, or concert.

I will explain why the best way to assess risk is to take a macro-perspective rather than a microscopic look at a given activity, event, or behavior. When evaluating the pros and cons of doing anything in our new normal, we also can't make decisions in a vacuum or a bubble—we need to be able to integrate numerous factors relating to our environment, pathogens (and not just the coronavirus), each other, and ourselves. These elements are not static; they are ever-changing. And we need to be able to change with them.

But it's not just about risk assessment—risk mitigation is just as important. In this chapter, I'll give you the tools to make informed decisions and take proactive steps to lower your chances of getting infected with COVID-19 (or any other contagious illness) in public places. All in all, it's about learning how to empower yourself to feel good about your choices to be in public and stay healthy and happy no matter what you choose to do.

HOW TO THINK LIKE A DOCTOR TO ASSESS YOUR SAFETY IN PUBLIC PLACES

Is it safe to do X, Y, or Z? is by far the most frequent question I've received from viewers, patients, family, and friends since the coronavirus outbreak began, but it's not an easy question to answer. What we know about the virus is continually evolving, along with guidelines from global, federal, state, local, and tribal officials. What's more, every situation is unique, and what going back to work looks like for someone in the service industry, for example, will likely be different from the guy or gal with an office job who doesn't have to regularly interact with the public.

For these reasons, instead of suggesting you memorize particulars about how the virus may or may not impact certain public places, I want to encourage you to do something I've advocated throughout this entire book: think like a doctor. If you adopt the mental process a doctor would use to assess each individual situation, you have the ability to make the best decisions for you and your family, based on the unique circumstances surrounding what you want to do, alongside your own personal risk factors and tolerance. And you will be able to do this for every situation that comes your way.

The first step in thinking like a doctor, then, is to evaluate everything we know about the situation and the inherent risk it poses. In today's new normal, we can distill situational risk of becoming infected with COVID-19 down to four major factors:

» **Time:** How long will you be at the public place? In general, any events that last longer than fifteen minutes require some safety scrutiny.

» **Place:** Will you be inside or outside? If inside, are there windows and doors that will or can be open? Or will there be adequate ventilation?

» **People:** How many people will be with you, approximately? Or how densely crowded will the place be? Is there a mask mandate that ensures everyone will be wearing a face covering?

» **Space:** How much space will there be between you and other people? Will you be seated or standing in one place for a duration of time or can you move about? In general, more space apart is safer than less space.

In addition to these four factors, there's also your city or state percent positivity rate, which reflects the percentage of people who test positive for coronavirus in your area. The percent positive isn't a total case count—instead, it indicates how widespread COVID-19 infection is in the area where testing is occurring. If your city or state has a percent positive rate of 1 percent or below, for example, your risk of contracting the coronavirus is relatively low—but it's not nonexistent. By comparison, the World Health

Organization advised governments in May 2020 to maintain a percent positive rate at or below 5 percent for at least two weeks before reopening. Many states, however, have not adhered to this suggestion and have remained opened with percent positives in the double digits. Whatever the case may be in your area, a high percent positivity is reason to avoid public places. But again, realize that there is still a risk of contracting COVID-19 if your state or city has a percent positive rate below 1 percent.

After you've assessed the total situational risk, including your area's percent positivity rate, the next step is to evaluate your physical risk factors in the situation. In the instance of COVID-19, physical risk depends on how old you are, how healthy you are, and whether you have any specific medical conditions that may make you more vulnerable to severe complications. To learn more about these conditions, see chapter 1.

Your degree of physical risk may also shape your degree of risk tolerance—another variable to evaluate when you're discerning whether it's safe for you to do X, Y, or Z. If you have multiple physical risk factors, for example, or live with someone who has multiple physical risk factors, your risk tolerance will likely be lower than someone who doesn't. Your risk tolerance may also be lower because you simply don't feel as comfortable as others in certain situations in our new normal. Just like fingerprints, everyone's risk tolerance is unique, as it should be—it never has or will be one size fits all. As we discussed in chapter 9, some people may be comfortable sky diving out of a plane while others wouldn't even step foot in a small plane, let alone jump out of one.

Recognize that your risk tolerance may also be tied to nonnegotiable risks—those activities you have to do in our new normal. For example, an essential worker may not want to take any additional risks by seeing a movie or eating at a restaurant because they're already interacting with the public every day. This is how I feel. Since I already see patients and go into the ABC studios, where I can't wear a mask while having my makeup done or when I'm on air, I'm selective about what other risks I'm willing to take. On the other hand, people who work from home may feel more comfortable introducing risk every now and then to eat out or go to the movies.

Finally, consider what all good doctors analyze about all our patients: the mental and emotional side. Ask yourself how important it is to you to do X, Y, or Z—mentally and emotionally. Personally, as much as I enjoy doing so, eating at a restaurant is not important to me, but getting a pedicure or having my hair done is. Both activities are part of my self-care and make me feel good. For others, going to church, seeing art, or traveling to an event is worth the risk these activities involve.

When people ask me if it's safe to do something, they often want to know if it's safe to do that activity as they would have in B.C. (before coronavirus) times. But you can't gauge the safety of any activity in our new normal using an old-normal filter—that's why we call it *the new normal*. So, if you're wondering whether it's safe to host a dinner party, for example, the answer would be no if you plan on sitting a bunch of unmasked people around a small table inside your home like we would have in 2019. But if you intend to hold a dinner party outside where you distance the chairs and everyone wears masks except while eating, then you can likely make it safe—or as safe as possible.

This last caveat is important: As you know, you can never remove risk entirely. When it comes to an infectious disease like COVID-19, whenever you have more than one person in a room, you have a risk. You can choose to live alone and never leave your house, but by doing so, you could also fall down the stairs, get struck by lightning, or develop heart disease—a real risk factor associated with social isolation. I'm not trying to scare you or be melodramatic, but I do want to remind you that perspective matters. In our new normal, we should keep living our lives, but simply try to do so as safely as possible.

IS IT SAFE TO GO BACK TO WORK?

We all have really different jobs, in really different job environments. Some people work in an office with ten people, others work in an office with a thousand people, and others don't work in an office at all but deal with the public all day. When we talk about whether it's safe to go back to work and/or how to lower your risk at work, the answer partly depends on your particular job. The other part of the answer doesn't, which is the part we'll talk about here.

To begin with, I can't tell you whether it's safe for you to go back to your work without knowing what you do for a living, how healthy and old you are, and the four factors we already outlined for situational risk: the time, place, people, and space of your work. In other words, how long will your workdays be? Will your environment be well-ventilated and/or can you open windows and doors? How many people will you be working with, and will they all be wearing masks? How densely populated is your working environment? I suggest you weigh these considerations alongside your own health, risk factors, and risk tolerance. At the same time, I realize many people don't have a choice whether they return to work. Either way, whether you're already back at work, have decided that you will go back to work, or have no choice in the matter, I suggest you do everything you can to make your working environment as safe as possible.

Before I went back to seeing patients in person at my medical practice in New Jersey, I intentionally strategized with my staff on how to make it as safe as possible. Sure, I had safety guidelines from the state, but guidelines are like medical textbooks: They're great to consult, but ultimately you have to diagnose and treat the patient or situation based on individual symptoms or signs. So before we reopened, I met with my clinical assistant, Ana, and my practice administrator, Carole, to come up with a plan to increase safety within the parameters of our practice without interfering with our quality of care. As it turns out, there were a number of small modifications we could make that have provided big benefits in the pandemic age.

Today, for example, we don't use a waiting room or reception area, but instead ask patients to wait in their cars until we're ready to call them by phone and escort them inside directly to an exam room. We also ask patients to fill out a questionnaire (with a disposable golf pencil!) to help assess whether they may have been exposed to COVID-19 after running through a list of questions with them by phone. (Our office is 99 percent paperless, but our patient software is not adaptable to online or mobile questionnaires.) Everyone wears a mask and we purposefully leave the door to the exam room open, along with windows when possible, to improve ventilation throughout the practice.

We take other precautions, too, like limiting how long I speak with new patients in my office and shortening the appointment time for existing patients. Before the pandemic, I typically spent one hour with new patients and thirty minutes with established patients. In our new normal, I have shortened those times considerably. These modifications don't reflect how I prefer to practice medicine, but I try to see both as necessary sacrifices. While I may be able to extend appointment time in the coming years, other modifications will remain in place for the foreseeable future. The pandemic has permanently altered many aspects of our world, so it's not surprising that going to work—or going to see the doctor, if you're one of my patients—has been permanently altered, too.

My return-to-work story is unique, as is everyone's, but it shows some of the universal truths we now have to contend with in our new normal. Here are some of the strategies I recommend to make work as safe as possible for everyone involved:

• **Start with words, then actions.** Talk with your employer first about what safety measures are in place. If you believe your company could be doing more, speak up—and don't worry about being the squeaky wheel. Health safety on the job has become the equivalent of sexual harassment in the workplace: If someone says they don't feel comfortable, your employer has a responsibility to do something about it.

• **Adhere to COVID-19 101.** Everyone should be doing the same things at work that they do everywhere else: Wear a mask. Respect each other's space. Wash your hands regularly. Just because you're spending up to eight hours at work doesn't mean you can pull down your mask—if anything, the longer you spend in one location, the more important it is to wear a mask over your nose and mouth.

• **Come in late or leave early.** Talk with your employer about staggering work hours to lower the number of people in an office or business at one time.

• **Avoid extra steps.** We've all heard that we should walk to a colleague's office instead of sending an email or calling in order to spend less time sitting. But in our new normal, the fewer face-to-face interactions you have, the safer it'll be for everyone. For extra steps, head outside and take a walk around the block.

• **Open windows and doors.** When possible, open windows to help ventilate rooms and reduce the risk of exposure to possible viral particles. Leaving doors open between rooms will also increase ventilation and airflow.

• **Drop the in-office coffee habit.** Common kitchens, coffee stations, and eating areas shouldn't exist in our new normal. If they do at your job, avoid them.

• **Give up being Mr. or Ms. Martyr.** I can't tell you how many times I've overheard people at work almost bragging about how sick they were the night before. I understand that some people don't get paid if they don't go to work and that others feel like they have too many responsibilities to stay home. Either way, no amount of money or number of responsibilities is a reason to endanger someone else's health. Admittedly, I used to be guilty of thinking I couldn't take a day off, but then I stayed home a few times and a shocking thing happened: The world continued to rotate on its axis. Yours will, too, I promise.

A Note to All Our Essential Workers

To all the grocery-store clerks, bus drivers, mail-delivery people, pharmacists, healthcare workers, restaurant staff, and other essential employees: You know who you are. America now knows just how essential you are and how risky your jobs can be, especially for many black and brown people, who are at a higher risk of being exposed and developing severe complications from COVID-19. I want to acknowledge that you didn't have control over when you went back to work and that many of you haven't been able to significantly reduce the number of risk factors you face while there. For all these reasons and much more, our country owes you a massive debt of gratitude. From Dr. Jennifer Ashton to you: Thank you.

IS IT SAFE TO TRAVEL?

People are eager to travel—I hear it every day from viewers, patients, family, and friends who want to know whether it's safe to fly, take a road trip, or stay at a hotel. Since every trip is unique to begin with, I suggest filtering your intended excursion through our four fundamental factors: time, place, people, and space.

» **Time:** How long will you be traveling for?

» **Place:** Are you traveling by air, car, train, or bus? And will you also be in an airport, train terminal, or bus station?

» **People:** Who will you be traveling with? For example, are you taking a cross-country drive with someone from your household or four friends from separate households? Will everyone be wearing masks or does your intended air/train/bus carrier have a good reputation for enforcing its mask policy?

» **Space:** How crowded will your means of travel be? Does your intended air/train/bus carrier limit capacity or have an open-seat policy?

Now, think about your destination. Are you traveling to a place with a high incidence of COVID-19 or other illnesses? Remember not to overlook other destination-specific ailments like traveler's diarrhea, which can be more of a likely risk than the coronavirus. Also, what will you do while you're there? For example, will you be camping in the woods with your family where you may be exposed to tick-borne illnesses like Lyme disease or babesiosis, or are you planning on sightseeing through a major city with thousands of other people? While many get hung up over fretting whether to fly or drive, the variables of your destination are just as important as how you'll get there.

The Truth About Air Travel

While many are fearful to fly, the truth about air travel in our new normal is that it may be one of the safest means of public transportation. While outbreaks of COVID-19 have happened from cruise ships, personal parties, and business conferences, there hasn't been one published report to date of an outbreak occurring from an airplane.

Air travel, in general, is also safer than taking a train or bus. Why? As Captain Tajer explained, commercial airplanes have HEPA air filters, which help to clean the cabin's air of particles the same size as, and even smaller than, the coronavirus.[1] HEPA filters also circulate air through the cabin once every several minutes, providing a degree of ventilation you won't usually find on trains, buses, or other forms of public transport.[2] Most airlines also have strict mandatory mask polices that are enforced by flight attendants (compared to trains or buses, where employees may not have the same oversight over passengers). Some airlines also block the sale of the middle seats on planes, which significantly helps reduce density and risk.

For these reasons, it's estimated that airline passengers have a 1 in 4,300 chance of catching COVID-19 during a two-hour flight if everyone is wearing masks, according to a study from MIT.[3] These odds drop considerably—to 1 in 7,700—on flights where the middle seat is left open.[4] Compare that to the 1 in 5,900 odds you have of catching COVID-19 by going about your daily business in the United States, according to the researchers. As for your odds of dying from COVID-19 if you do become infected with the virus on a plane, the MIT study put the risk of death at 1 in 400,000 for full flights and 1 in 600,000 if the middle seat is left open.[5]

Bottom line: You can feel pretty safe about flying in our new normal. You can also increase the safety of your trip by following these tips:

» Choose an airline that blocks the sale of middle seats.
» Book a window seat to keep your distance from people moving up and down the aisle.
» Check in online to minimize personal contact.

» Immediately upon boarding, wipe down the tray table, armrests, and anything else you might touch, primarily to prevent the spread of other infectious illnesses like the flu and norovirus.

» Consider wearing eye protection. While it's not an official CDC recommendation, Dr. Anthony Fauci and other infectious disease experts say wearing some kind of eye protection like eyeglasses, reading glasses, sunglasses, or face shields can help shield the mucous membranes in your eyes from possible exposure to viral particles. While you don't need to wear eye protection in your day-to-day life, I'd suggest adopting the habit whenever you'll be inside an enclosed space for a prolonged period of time. Just remember that wearing eye protection like a face shield is NOT a substitute for a mask.

Of course, a plane isn't the only space you'll be inside during an air-travel trip. The good news is that most major airports are big, and you can easily find space at least six feet away from others—something that's a little more difficult to come by in busy train stations and bus terminals. Remember to always wear your mask and stay moving to prevent breathing in the same air from one person for a sustained period of time.

One advantage to traveling by plane in our new normal: Fewer people may get sick from colds, stomach bugs, the flu, and other infectious disease, thanks to new mask policies and less crowded flights.

The Safest Way to Go: Your Own Automobile

The safest way to travel anywhere in our new normal is by yourself in your own car, where you can't possibly breathe in anyone else's respiratory droplets. That said, few people take long road trips all alone—we like to go with family and friends.

Perhaps unsurprisingly, the safest person to road trip with in a pandemic is someone you live with. But doing so isn't a fail-safe. Because you'll be spending hours in a very small space with the same person, you'll be exposed to their respiratory droplets directly and for a longer period of time than you may be by going about your daily life together in the same household. For these reasons, you may want to both consider getting tested for COVID-19 or quarantining at home for fourteen days before you jump in the car together for hours on end. If you choose to ride with someone outside your household or immediate pandemic pod, I suggest everyone get tested or self-quarantine for two weeks (or as long as possible) prior to the trip.

If you want to increase everyone's safety while in the car, keep windows rolled down as often as possible and wear masks. If you stop for gas or food, be sure everyone washes their hands thoroughly before getting back into the car.

Hotels: Probably Safer Than You Think

A lot of people have asked me whether it's safe to stay at a hotel or a motel. Personally and professionally, I believe the answer is yes. While we don't understand how easily the coronavirus can or can't be spread through heating, ventilation, and air-conditioning (HVAC) systems (see box on page 219), it appears right now that ventilation systems don't pose a significant threat of COVID-19 transmission.

Another reason that hotels may be safe: You're likely staying by yourself or with one other person. While a hotel room isn't equivalent to a negative pressure room inside a hospital, you're still in relative isolation. The room was cleaned beforehand, and you have the ability to take additional disinfection measures by wiping down high-touch surfaces when you first arrive. Better still, if possible, open the windows as soon as you check in and head out for a walk while fresh air circulates through the room. If you feel uncomfortable or aren't able to take a walk, wear a mask for the first few hours to prevent breathing in the respiratory droplets of the cleaning staff (who were most likely wearing masks) or the room's past occupants (who likely checked out hours before you arrived).

All in all, staying at a hotel may be safer than staying the night with friends or family who aren't part of your pandemic pod. When you stay with other people, it's very difficult to avoid breathing in their respiratory droplets. Not only will you be immersed in the same indoor air for hours at a time, you'll also not be able to wear a mask while eating, drinking, and sleeping. You also may have less control over whether you can open windows and doors.

If you choose to stay at a hotel, keep in mind that it's not just the room, but the entire hotel that will be part of your experience. Opt for contactless check-in and checkout, avoid getting into elevators with other people, and stay away from breakfast buffets and common coffee areas.

Can COVID-19 Be Spread Through HVAC Systems?

All the infectious disease experts I've spoken with say they don't believe at this time that the spread of COVID-19 through heating, ventilation, and air-conditioning (HVAC) systems poses a significant risk. While studies suggest the virus can survive in air ducts, detection doesn't mean infection, and there's inconclusive evidence showing whether the disease can be readily spread through HVAC systems.[6] HVAC systems by nature remove particles and exchange indoor air for outdoor air, which may even help reduce the risk of COVID-19 spread.[7] To increase the efficacy of your HVAC system in pandemic times, the World

Health Organization recommends boosting the percentage of outdoor air it uses, along with its filtration potential.[8] The WHO also suggests running an HVAC system for two hours before or after occupancy. For this reason, you may want to consider switching on the heat or A/C when you check in and leave your hotel.

IS IT SAFE TO GO TO THE GYM?

Because you know I love the gym, you probably won't be surprised to learn that this topic has been a HUGE question mark for me. I've missed my regular gym routine every single day since the pandemic began, as have many fellow exercise enthusiasts. You might not love to work out, but for many people, not being able to go to a gym or take a fitness class has created a significant amount of physical and psychological stress.

Despite my mental and emotional distress, I haven't jumped at the chance to lift weights inside a club or take a spin class in the city with friends. Gyms have always been prime places for infectious illness, given the number of people sweating, breathing hard, touching equipment, and also touching their faces inside a confined space. They're often crowded, and people tend to stay there for up to an hour or more at one time. Add in a contagious respiratory virus that's easier to contract through forceful breathing, and you can understand why I—and many others—have thought twice about this popular pastime.

But everyone is different, and just because I may not feel comfortable working out inside a gym doesn't mean you won't be— and can't stay safe while doing it. To assess your risk in using a gym, I'd start by evaluating your physical health. If you're in a high-risk group for severe complications with COVID-19 or live with someone who is, I might find alternative ways to work out that don't involve an indoor environment (see chapter five for ideas).

If you're not high-risk, the answer of whether it's safe for you to work out inside a gym depends partly on the facility. Some gyms require reservations or limit capacity; others may also do temperature checks and/or have members complete questionnaires about possible COVID-19 exposure before working out. Some facilities also open windows or have open-air roofs for increased ventilation. Many have a strict mask policy—whether employees enforce it depends on your individual facility—space equipment more than six feet apart, and routinely disinfect shared areas. The more measures a gym takes, the safer it will be for you to go.

That said, I would avoid taking an indoor fitness class like spin or yoga with other people. These types of classes typically involve a number of people working out in a small, enclosed room for up to an hour at a time, breathing the same air. In an indoor class, you have sustained exposure to the respiratory droplets of others, which is the primary way COVID-19 (and many other contagious respiratory illnesses) is spread. Consider taking these classes outdoors or online if offered.

To further lower your risk when going to the gym, consider these additional tips:

» Only frequent fitness facilities that offer a reservation policy or limit total capacity. The fewer people inside a gym, the lower your risk of possible infectious illness.

» If you want to work out at a gym without a reservation policy, go during off-peak hours or call in advance to make sure the facility is not crowded.

» Stay as far away as possible from other people while working out, especially if you or someone else is inhaling or exhaling forcefully. Ten feet is better than six feet when people are breathing heavily, but six feet is also better than two feet.

» Don't touch your face. This is easy to forget in day-to-day life and even easier when you're physically exerting yourself.

» Wipe down all equipment before and after each use. Don't assume the facility's employees or other guests will do it for you.

» Always wear a mask. I know it's tempting to remove it when you're working out, but you shouldn't, especially when you're participating in a high-risk activity like exercising inside with others.

IS IT SAFE TO EAT AT RESTAURANTS?

Before the pandemic, I loved eating out at all the amazing restaurants in New York City and Boston and would do so regularly. Today, though, I don't eat at any restaurants, whether the tables are inside or outside. While I commiserate immensely with the restaurant industry and try to still support them by ordering takeout and delivery, I simply don't feel comfortable sitting within six feet of someone else for ninety minutes at a time while we both have our masks down to eat and drink. Given the fact I see patients and work in an office every day, it's not an additional risk I'm willing to take.

How do you know whether eating at a restaurant is a risk you can take? Perhaps no other activity is more apt for our four factors of time, place, people, and space than dining with others:

» **Time:** How long will you be at the restaurant?

» **Place:** Will you be eating outside or inside? If inside, does the restaurant have open windows or will the front door be ajar?

» **People:** How many people will be inside the restaurant? Or how many will be in your immediate vicinity if you're eating outside?

» **Space:** Is the restaurant large with high ceilings or is it a small room? Are the tables at least six feet apart? Is it a noisy place where people may be talking loudly, thereby exhaling more particles into the air?

When you assess these factors, you might decide that eating inside at a restaurant is one of the riskier things you can do right now, especially since people don't (and really can't) wear masks while dining and drinking.

Another way to look at it: What is the worst-case scenario that can happen if you do eat at a restaurant? Let's say you're seated next to someone with COVID-19 who isn't wearing a mask. Let's also say the airflow inside the restaurant or the breeze if you're outside is just right that it directs his or her respiratory droplets toward you for a period of time. Let's also assume you're not wearing a mask either because you're eating and drinking. That's a high risk of exposure.

I want to be clear about one thing: There's nothing a restaurant can do to make your experience safer other than space tables far apart, put plexiglass or plastic barriers between outdoor tables, require masks, and open windows and doors when allowing customers to dine inside. (Aerosol scientists say that plexiglass barriers at best are helpful only against large droplets and at worst do nothing against smaller aerosol particles.) Otherwise, if someone walks into a restaurant with COVID-19 and takes off his or her mask for two hours to eat and drink, I don't care how far apart the tables are or how amazing the ventilation is, that's a significant risk of exposure. The fact that your server is wearing a mask shouldn't give you a false sense of security: Waiters and waitresses visit tables for no more than a few minutes at a time. Instead, it's everyone else seated at the restaurant whom you have to worry about.

Eating outdoors is definitely safer when it comes to COVID-19 transmission, just like all outdoor activities are. But keep in mind that you can still sit in direct airflow of someone with the virus for up to several hours at a time while neither of you are wearing masks.

In short, there are no easy answers when it comes to eating out at restaurants. I encourage you to consider if the reward is worth the risk. When you do so, try (as hard as it is) to separate evidence from emotion: Most of us, me included, would love to be eating out as often as we could, but that doesn't mean we should be.

One thing you can feel good about if you do decide to eat out: There's absolutely no evidence of COVID-19 infection because a server breathed on your food or carried a dish through air with viral particles. There's also no evidence that you can contract the virus from food that's been handled by someone infected with COVID-19. Again, this is a respiratory virus, and the primary means of transmission is through respiratory droplets in the air.

Is It Safe to Use a Public Restroom?

Public restrooms are petri dishes, as most people know. They're small enclosed spaces with a lot of high-touch surfaces. What's more, the virus has been detected in urine and stool and has been shown to aerosolize into the air when the toilet flushes. That said, if you have to use a public bathroom, you shouldn't feel afraid. Wear a mask, minimize the time you spend there, and wash your hands well before you leave. Remember, too, that you likely didn't think twice about using a public restroom before the coronavirus pandemic, even though it harbored (and still does) *plenty* of nasty illnesses like rotavirus and norovirus, both of which can be spread through contaminated feces.

IS IT SAFE TO GO TO THE SALON?

Before the coronavirus outbreak began, going to the salon was an integral part of my self-care. I've always found it relaxing to have my hair done or get a manicure or pedicure—they're activities that make me feel like I'm taking care of myself and nurturing myself. (Plus, it helps me not scare my patients or our ABC viewers!) But in our new normal, I've had to rethink whether these activities are worth the risk. In doing so, I've explored whether there are viable alternatives to being in a public place with other people. I've done this with other activities in this chapter, too. For example, instead of eating at a restaurant, I can get takeout—and for me, that's a very viable alternative with a much, much lower risk.

But with salon services, I haven't found many viable alternatives. While I've learned to take care of my own fingernails and live without manicures, I can't seem to maintain my feet no matter how hard I try—these babies need professional help. And doing my own hair isn't really an option because I'm on TV every day. For these reasons, I've made the decision to go to salons occasionally to have my hair done and get a pedicure.

That said, I'm not running into every hair or nail salon I see in the city whenever my hair looks dull or my toes seem a little ragged (despite the fact there are hair and nail salons on almost every city block and my toes always seem to look a little ragged). Instead, I try to be selective about when, where, and how often I go.

Whether you're already at the salon regularly or thinking about a visit, here are the tips I use to make the experience safer:

» Rethink how often you go. Can you use a special product to touch up your hair color or your manicure at home to help it last longer? Could you try an at-home facial or beg your spouse for a shoulder massage? As a bonus, the longer you go between appointments, the more money you'll save.

» Call salons in advance to find out what safety measures are in place. Some offer plastic or plexiglass barriers between guests and/or between you and the nail technician. (But note that some aerosol scientists consider these barriers "useless," since particles can go around and above them.) Additionally, some businesses do temperature checks and/or limit guest capacity. The more safety measures in place, the lower your possible risk.

» Book an appointment during off-peak hours if your schedule allows. Even if a salon limits capacity, you're more likely to encounter fewer people on a Monday morning than a Friday or Saturday afternoon.

» Don't wait inside before your appointment. Ask the receptionist, stylist, or technician to call you when they're ready for you.

» Ask your masseuse, facialist, stylist, or technician to open windows and doors to increase ventilation. Most businesses are happy to comply, especially if you explain it's safer for everyone.

» Wear a mask and eye protection.

» Use contactless payment like Venmo or Apple Pay whenever possible and leave cash tips in envelopes.

IS IT SAFE TO GO TO HOUSES OF WORSHIP?

For centuries, houses of worship have helped fuel the spread of infectious disease—and the coronavirus pandemic is no different. Churches in South Korea, for example, helped spark the country's initial outbreak, along with a second wave months later.[9] A church service in Arkansas sickened thirty-five congregants, three who died, at the very beginning of the pandemic in the United States.[10] As of July 2020, 650 cases of COVID-19 had been linked to nearly forty religious services and events nationwide.[11] What's more, published reports suggest that some infections occurred in houses of worship where congregants wore masks and followed social distancing guidelines.[12]

What makes houses of worships so risky in our new normal? Churches, mosques, and synagogues by nature bring a lot of people together in one small space at the same time. They often include loud sermons and singing, both of which have been shown to transmit more viral particles. In addition, people often hug, kiss, or shake hands at religious services, even in our new normal when doing so is not advised.

When you apply our four factors—time, place, people, and space—the answers often stack up that a religious service will be moderate to high risk. Most services are at least an hour long and are held indoors, often in poorly ventilated spaces, where people are often singing, forcefully projecting viral particles into the air. For these reasons, epidemiologists have ranked religious services as high risk.[13]

I understand that religious services are a fundamental part of many people's lives—and giving them up, for many, is simply not an option. If you choose to attend a religious service, acknowledge the risk and wear a mask and eye protection. Find a service that enforces a mask policy and social distancing measures. If you can, choose a service that doesn't feature singing and/or prioritizes silent prayer over loud oratory. Don't share hymnals or other worship items. Finally, speak with church or synagogue leaders about opening windows and doors, if they aren't already, even in colder months.

If you don't have to attend in person, consider virtual services, which is how I've chosen to worship since the pandemic began. Since many services are now live-streamed, you can feel like you're right inside your church, synagogue, or mosque, but without any of the risk. If you miss interacting with other congregants or spiritual leaders, attend an outdoor function like a church picnic instead.

IS IT SAFE TO GO TO MUSEUMS, THEATERS, AND CONCERTS?

First, some good news: No other category in this chapter may provide more safe, viable alternatives to in-person events than the arts. Museums, theaters, dance companies, Broadway performers, musicians, filmmakers, and other artists or art organizations have all stepped up in our new normal to offer a ton of online exhibits, shows, and performances. Virtual is obviously not the same as seeing these things live in person, but it can certainly help scratch the itch while keeping you and your family safe. Similarly, you can now find lots of outdoor exhibits and performances, which are much safer than their indoor counterparts.

Your next safest bet if you're craving a culture shot may be to go to a museum. In a museum, you can move from place to place, finding areas that are less crowded and also avoiding breathing in the same air of the same people for an extended period of time. There's almost never any loud talking or singing in a museum by rule, and you can easily choose to visit during off-peak hours. Personally, I find museums magical at night, which is usually when they're the least crowded.

Theaters are trickier—and potentially riskier. In a theater, you're sitting in the same spot for up to three hours at a time, and you might be in direct airflow of someone with COVID-19, even if they're more than six feet away from you. Everyone should be wearing masks, however, which makes the activity hypothetically safer than dining at a restaurant. That said, I'd avoid going to a theater that sells food or drinks so that no one is pulling down his or her mask to munch or sip. Call in advance to make sure the theater you want to visit has closed its concession stand for this reason.

Of all the arts, live concerts may be the riskiest in our new normal because, similar to houses of worship, many feature loud singing and talking. Concerts held with theater seating carry the same risks as regular theaters, while floor seats include the very real possibility that people won't remain standing at least six feet apart for the entire show. If you're craving live music, look for outdoor venues where the risk of transmission is much lower. Some famous concerts have been held outside at various amphitheaters and can be a safer alternative, especially if you wear a mask and follow social distancing measures.

Using the information in this chapter, you can feel empowered to make the best decisions for you and your family about how to stay safe in public places. While you can never negate the risk of getting sick from COVID-19 or any other infectious illness if it exists in your town or city, you can learn how to navigate shared spaces more safely. You can also make decisions about what you do and don't do in public spaces from a place of knowledge rather than one of assumption, misperception, or fear. Remember that COVID-19 will be with us for years to come. Learning to live safely with the virus—and any other pathogen that might come our way—while continuing to enjoy your life will allow you to stay happy and healthy in our new normal.

CHAPTER 11

Silver Linings

There's been no shortage of silver linings born out of the coronavirus outbreak. You've likely heard about some of them, if you haven't experienced a few yourself: families spending more time together, friends reconnecting, everyone cooking more, millions finally finding time to slow down, take a breath, and discover new passions that have helped transform their lives or livelihood.

If you've lost a loved one, you may have a hard time finding any bright breaks in the clouds—and understandably so. The same is true for anyone who's lost their job, home, or business. Nothing can compensate for these losses, I realize. But without any loss at all, silver linings couldn't exist. By definition, it takes some dark clouds for a sun-edged periphery to appear, which is where *silver lining* gets its name. And looking for the silver linings is certainly better than remaining in the gloom without any sun to illuminate the dark.

In this chapter, I don't want to twist anyone's arm to try to find a silver lining. And I don't want to retell the personal stories of the pandemic's positive outcomes, as amazing as they are, because they're unique to each person. What I want to do is share with you the silver lining lessons that the pandemic taught us. What are the silver lining lessons? They're the tough realities that we learned during the outbreak, and while they may have been difficult to grasp, we now have an opportunity to take advantage of the adversity and leverage of these lessons in order to improve ourselves and our lives.

Let me tell you what happened to me. Several months into the initial outbreak, I was on set preparing to tape *GMA3* when I looked over at Amy Robach, the show's co-anchor and my friend for almost ten years—as long as I've been at ABC News. By this point in the pandemic, we had been working overtime for weeks, along with dozens of others at ABC News, to report on the virus, despite what was happening all around us in New York City and the rest of the country and world.

As I glanced at Amy, the slide show of our friendship flashed through my mind. I was with her in a mobile mammogram truck, for example, when she had her first mammogram that detected her breast cancer. Years later, she was one of the first people at work whom I told I was getting a divorce from my then-husband, Rob. Several months after, she became one of my rocks at work when Rob ended his life. We were also both shocked by the death of one of the *Good Morning America* camera operators due to COVID-19. She constantly inspired in the early outbreak and motivated me, both professionally and personally.

Despite these hardships, there we were, still alive and on set, covering the pandemic for a show seen across the country by millions of people. But now, it wasn't only Amy suffering with breast cancer or me suffering through the death of my ex-husband—it was all of us, everyone on set and everyone watching from home, suffering through a profound and universal hardship. And yet there we all still were—not only surviving but functioning and even stepping up in ways we never thought possible.

When I look back at the initial outbreak, I still can't believe it. Day after day for months on end, I went on air for up to thirteen hours a day, processing, analyzing, and integrating massive amounts of medical news. I did it because I had to—I had no other choice. I stepped up for myself, my ABC News work family, and the job that I love. I stepped up for the up to 11 million viewers who relied on me for accurate and honest information. And I stepped up because I knew that, among the millions of viewers, there were two people always watching me: my children. And there was no way I was going to let them down.

While your circumstances are undoubtedly different, your story is the same as mine: You stepped up. We all did. You stayed strong in one way or another, whether it was for yourself, your family, your colleagues, your neighbors, or simply the strangers you encountered on the street or in the stores every day. We all stepped up in our own way, and as a result, every single one of us is more resilient now than we were in December 2019.

While other major crises—wars, famine, natural disasters, 9/11—have shown us how much strength some people have, the coronavirus outbreak has proven the power inside us all. Unlike other crises, the pandemic has been global, not regional or specific to a certain city or country. Additionally, there's been no way for anyone to escape it—you couldn't hop on an airplane and fly out of the danger zone, hide out in remote areas of the country (there have been viral hot spots in rural regions, after all), or buy your way into a guarantee against infection.

Perhaps most profoundly, the pandemic has lasted for more than a year—not days or weeks—battering and burnishing each of us over time. This, in turn, has caused a tiny rock of resiliency to form inside us all, not unlike a precious diamond that won't weaken or fade with time. To me, this universal uptick in individual resiliency is one of the biggest silver lining lessons out of the entire pandemic: Hard times create little stones of strength inside everyone who endures them.

We've learned other silver lining lessons, too. Many, at first blush, can appear more like negative outcomes than positive developments. But in each of these difficult lessons, there's an opportunity to leverage the hardship to improve ourselves and our lives.

It reminds me of what happens with some of my patients. In my twenty years as a doctor, I've had to tell many the unimaginable: They have cancer, for example, or they've tested positive for HIV; their unborn baby has died; they won't be able to have children. These are difficult diagnoses to live through, but in some patients, the hardship unlocks something amazing inside them. Months later, these patients come back and say to me, *You know what, Dr. Ashton? Getting cancer* (or X, Y, or Z ailment) *was the best thing that ever happened me.* They then proceed to tell me how they felt like they were running on a treadmill before they got sick, but that their diagnosis forced them to get off, learn to savor the moment at hand, start living life again, and prioritize what's important.

This is not an unusual story—you might have heard something similar from someone you know. Or maybe you've even experienced it yourself. Either way, not every patient can see, let alone leverage, the silver lining lesson in a difficult diagnosis. But the silver lining lessons always exist, and it's up to you to leverage what you've learned and transform an unfortunate situation into a remarkable opportunity.

The new normal has changed how we all look at silver linings. While they've traditionally been things we recognize only in hindsight, the pandemic has forced us to look for silver linings right now in real time—both the duration and disruptive nature of our new normal don't give us the luxury of hindsight. We need to be able to spot the breaks through the clouds while the storm is still occurring. Doing so allows us not only to stay sane but also to learn the lessons that the silver linings can teach us so we can build more resilience to weather the storm even longer.

For the first part of this chapter, I want to share with you the silver lining lessons that we can all use to improve ourselves and our health. In the second half of the chapter, I want to share with you the pandemic's silver lining lessons that I believe we can use to improve medicine and the future of healthcare for everyone. I'm not talking only about healthcare as it relates to countries or hospital systems—I'm talking about the healthcare for YOU and your family.

SILVER LINING LESSONS FOR LIFE

Hardships can prepare ordinary people for extraordinary things, especially if you take the time to acknowledge what you're been through and consciously leverage what you've learned to make yourself healthier and happier. These are not abstract lessons we've learned during the pandemic but real, tangible truths to put into practice if we choose to. Here are four ways to do that and make the most of the difficulties we've all been through.

Silver Lining Lesson #1: We're All Responsible for Our Own Health

The coronavirus pandemic revealed a fundamental truth about the human condition that many have never had to face: Ultimately, each of us is responsible for our own health and well-being. The pandemic proved that institutions can't necessarily save us—or the government, technology, and medicine can't always prevent or defeat misfortune. Instead, it's up to each of us to assume control over the fate of our own bodies and well-being. In other words, individual health starts and ends with one person: the same one we see in the mirror every day.

This may be a hard truth to face, but it's an important and empowering one. Once you accept that you're ultimately responsible for you, you can assume ownership of your own well-being. Those who have done so in our new normal have lost weight, addressed chronic conditions like diabetes, started exercising again, finally found the impetus to treat a mental-health condition, or wrestled back control of another area of their health or happiness.

Taking control of our personal well-being also means learning the basics about when to go to the emergency room, what medications we may need and why, how to interpret medical news, and how to make good decisions—or find the right doctors who can help us make good decisions—about our own health.

Throughout this book, I've worked to show you what we can do to better adapt to our new normal in order to improve our health and happiness and become more self-sufficient and resilient. Instead of letting a virus decide that we can't exercise, for example, because it's not safe to be in a gym, we can come up with creative solutions to stay fit on our own. Instead of letting irrational fears about a pathogen prevent us from living life fully, we can educate ourselves about the disease and how to protect ourselves. Instead of refusing to travel or eat out, we can learn how to assess our own risks and make safer decisions for ourselves and everyone around us.

In many ways, our new normal has given us a do-it-yourself attitude about our own well-being. We now DIY exercise, for example, and DIY risk assessment to determine what's safe and not safe. We DIY our own meals, with more people cooking at home more often, and without a fixed schedule, many of us DIY our own sleep. We've had to DIY travel, work, and even our children's education in many instances, and with our social options so limited, we've been forced to DIY fun. Perhaps most important, we've had to step up and DIY our physical and emotional well-being. Now, as aspects of our old culture begin to return, I encourage you to retain this sense of self-sufficiency and resiliency.

Dr. Jen's Rx: It's a beautiful thing to learn and accept that it's ultimately up to us to make ourselves healthy and whole—physically, mentally, and emotionally. DIY wellness in the pandemic era is more than just useful; it can also be empowering and transformative.

Silver Lining Lesson #2: This Moment Is All We Have

The pandemic has exposed us all to a prolonged period of uncertainty that's unprecedented in recent human history. Safety guidelines and regulations have changed frequently. Borders, businesses, and schools have closed and reopened at a moment's notice. No one has been able to say when it would be safe to do certain activities, when there'd be a vaccine, or when life would "go back to normal." Instead, we've had to live each day in flux. This uncertainty has been a curse in many ways, but ultimately, it's a gift: When you can't look ahead to the future, you have to slow down and look at the here and now.

For many people, including me, it's not easy to live in the present. Before the pandemic, I was always going a hundred miles per hour, from the time I woke up in the morning to the moment I climbed into bed at night. Throughout my life, I've enjoyed being busy—I like the challenge, the energy, and the adrenaline it brings. I enjoyed thinking of and working toward a future goal, plan, or dream. Psychologically, being busy makes me feel good about myself, as though I'm hurtling through life full of productivity and intention.

But the pandemic has forced us all to slow down, me included. It's caused us to stop living life like we're hurtling along or running on a treadmill—that's a luxury we simply no longer have. Like some of my patients who receive a frightening medical diagnosis, we've been forced to hit the pause button. And by doing so, we've been given the opportunity to slow down, stop, and finally take the time to savor each and every moment.

Think about it. Before the pandemic, our collective calendars were jammed with work, school, travel, family, and social obligations and events. But when the outbreak began, we had no other choice but to cancel, postpone, or indefinitely delay almost every activity. In our new normal, we still can't plan for the future. What can we do? We can choose to live in the moment. That's not a comfortable way to subsist for many, but life begins outside our comfort zone.

For me, one of the biggest silver lining lessons is that it's okay not to plan each and every hour. We don't need to nor can we always schedule out what will happen next month, next week, or even the next day. All we have is today, this hour, this second. When we make the conscious decision to focus on what we have, we choose the ability to be truly happy, right here and now.

Dr. Jen's Rx: If we've learned anything from the coronavirus outbreak, it's that life can change drastically and inconceivably at the drop of a hat—or the discovery of a new disease. As our calendars and schedules begin to fill up, remember to enjoy what we can have right now.

Silver Lining Lesson #3: Some Things Matter More Than Others

Close your eyes and think about what your life was like in December 2019. What was important to you back then? Perhaps you were excited about a holiday party, finding the perfect gift for a family member or friend, or taking a winter vacation somewhere. Now think about what's important to you today. Maybe you're now focused on just getting back into the office, finding a new job, or being with your family in any way you can, vacation or not.

Many people's priorities have shifted as a result of our new normal. It's another advantage of being forced to slow down and finally stop: You can take stock of what's around you and realize what you do and don't want or need. The trivial fades into the background, and the truly important emerges as our main focus.

The pandemic has certainly helped me reevaluate what really matters. I've realized, for example, that I'm no longer willing to live in a different city from my boyfriend, especially if another pandemic prevents us from being together in person. We're now making modifications that we would never have considered if the coronavirus outbreak hadn't occurred. For this, I'm grateful that I was forced to recognize my priorities and take proactive steps to emphasize what's important.

Similar scenarios have played out in the lives and minds of millions of others around the world. Some people have realized that their families or friends matter more than the things they own, places they go, or jobs they have. Others no longer feel comfortable being a plane ride away from their families. Some want to make it possible for older parents or relatives to live with them if and when the next pandemic occurs.

In addition to relationships, the pandemic has shifted priorities for many about what they really want to do, whether professionally or personally. Some have realized that life is too short to work a job they don't love or have to wait to take a trip of a lifetime. Others have decided that they'd rather live a simpler life outside of the city. And almost all of us have reprioritized the importance of good health.

Dr. Jen's Rx: Don't lose sight of your pandemic priorities as life gets busy again. Focusing on what really matters, including family, friends, a fulfilling career, and good health, is imperative to being happy and healthy.

Silver Lining Lesson #4: It Could Be Worse

Whenever I've had to deliver an alarming diagnosis, I always let patients take a minute before I tell them how much worse it could be. For example, someone might have cancer, but at least they don't have stage IV cancer. Or if they do have stage IV cancer, I remind them how lucky they are to have access to quality healthcare or nearby family or friends who can help take care of them. I don't bring up the bright side to minimize what they're going through. But I know it helps people to put their diagnosis into perspective and shift focus from the things they've lost to what they already have. This way, they can replace feelings of fear, anxiety, and loneliness with feelings of gratitude.

During the pandemic, I tried to find perspective as often as I could so I could tap into new ways to be grateful. When my brother was diagnosed with COVID-19, for example, I told myself how thankful I was that he had access to some of the best care in the world. When he ended up showing symptoms, I reminded myself how grateful I was that he wasn't in the hospital or intubated. Putting things into perspective didn't erase my concern, but it helped me stay positive and weather adversity with strength and resilience. (After two weeks, my brother made a full recovery and has not manifested any long-haul symptoms, thankfully.)

This is an incredible silver lining lesson of our new normal: The pandemic has reminded many that we always have the choice. We can choose to dwell on what we've lost or flip it around and focus on what we've gained. This isn't easy, especially if you've suffered a terrible loss, but it can help you find resiliency in our new normal and be better prepared for whatever happens next.

Maybe you lost your job in the pandemic, for example, but perhaps you can be grateful that you didn't get sick with COVID-19—or if you did, that you were lucky enough to survive. If your relationship with your spouse or romantic partner has taken a hit in our new normal, that could be a good thing because it's helped you identify issues you needed to address—or maybe it will help you move on to find a more sustainable relationship in the future.

In short, there's always a bright side. And finding and focusing on the silver linings in our new normal can help you be grateful, develop more resiliency, and find a deeper sense of happiness.

Dr. Jen's Rx: While it can be easy to get tunnel vision during a crisis and dwell on how bad you may have it, try to put your new normal into perspective. It could always be worse. Replace feelings of fear, anxiety, or stress with gratitude whenever you can.

SILVER LINING LESSONS FOR MEDICINE

Just like there are silver lining lessons for each of us in our new normal, the pandemic has also taught the world of healthcare a few things that can and hopefully will reshape medicine for the better. While the full extent of these lessons are still to be seen, medicine is already changing to some degree because of what we've learned in the relatively short time since the COVID-19 crisis began. Similar to silver linings in our personal lives, silver linings in medicine are things that, on some level, healthcare professionals have known have been issues for years. But these last few months have reframed the importance and the urgency of these issues. And now that the stakes are clear, we as doctors and individuals have a chance to leverage these silver linings to improve our ability to help people.

Here are seven specific silver lining lessons that I believe have the power to overhaul how we handle the next pandemic and treat patients more safely and effectively for years to come.

Silver Lining Medical Lesson #1: Things Grow Stronger When You Integrate

Hospitals and medical centers regularly practice response drills. It's clinical medicine 101. No one wants to be doing a procedure for the first time or having to wing it when an emergency strikes. In medicine, if you don't practice something, you can't execute it. Simply put, drills save lives.

One of the best examples of this kind of medical preparedness happened within minutes of the Orlando Pulse nightclub shooting—the deadliest mass shooting in U.S. history when it occurred in 2016. I covered the story for ABC News and can tell you, as a fellow doctor, the response by Orlando Regional Medical Center (ORMC), located just three blocks away from Pulse, was absolutely phenomenal. Within forty-two minutes, ORMC received thirty-eight victims with gunshot wounds, most patients coming in after two in the morning when the ER was already on lockdown due to an active shooter situation in the area. Over the course of the next twenty-four hours, surgical teams at ORMC performed twenty-nine operations and saved forty of the forty-nine victims brought into the ER. Doctors there were able to do this only because ORMC, as the sole level one trauma center in all of central Florida, had drilled for this kind of scenario for years.

Similarly, when the coronavirus outbreak first impacted areas like New York City, many hospitals were prepared for an influx of patients because they'd rehearsed many times over. But individual hospital preparedness wasn't the problem. The problem instead was that the city—and the United States as a whole—had never prepared as one integrated medical community for a mass influx of patients across multiple hospitals.

Drills work in medicine—we knew that long before the coronavirus outbreak began. What the pandemic showed us is that we need to drill for medical emergencies at the city, county, state, and even national levels. We can and should expand the scale of our ready response exponentially, which many doctors (myself included) hope will happen before the next health crisis hits. We can no longer operate in a silo of one medical center or hospital— we need to shift our paradigm from hospitals thinking we're the whole team to one in which we realize we are part of a much larger team. If we do this, we have the potential to respond to the next pandemic swiftly and far more effectively.

Silver Lining Medical Lesson #2: We Need More Health Research on Race

Weeks into the coronavirus outbreak, we realized that COVID-19 was killing a disproportionate number of black and brown people. Yet by July 2020, the CDC was tracking race and ethnicity in only approximately 45 percent of all COVID-19 cases. That's not acceptable and they recognized that. While the organization was taxed in many ways, it should not have been difficult for the CDC to require all states to forward data on virus deaths and hospitalizations with race and ethnicity defined for every single patient.

What the pandemic has shown us once again is that we need more data about why some diseases occur at a higher rate among black and brown people. Some of this has to do with access to quality healthcare, but that's only part of the story. If you compare African American patients with health insurance to Caucasian people with health insurance, there is a greater incidence of disease in blacks, despite similar socioeconomic variables. Bottom line: Black and brown people represent unique populations with unique medical risks, and we need to tailor our healthcare system to meet these unique risks.

Time has run out on the need of public health agencies to address disparities in disease as they relate to race and ethnicity. We've known for years that we need more research in areas of race and pathology, but the pandemic has pushed the issue to the edge. Too many black and brown people lost their lives to COVID-19. If there's any silver lining lesson in this incredible loss, it's that their deaths don't have to be in vain.

Silver Lining Medical Lesson #3: World Health Matters

Over the last twenty years, the United States has watched from afar as other areas of the world have battled devasting outbreaks of infectious diseases like SARS, MERS, bird flu, yellow fever, Ebola, and Zika. While America has experienced isolated cases of some of these illnesses, we've remained largely U.S.-centric, not only immune from major flare-ups but also resistant to react to medical crises in other countries.

What the coronavirus pandemic has shown us, however, is that pathogens truly don't care whether you're in a developing country or the so-called First World. The misperception that somehow the United States can isolate and continue to remain immune to infectious illness is gone. The silver lining lesson here is that the United States should take a greater interest in global health.

Part of this is self-serving, of course: After seeing how quickly and pervasively the coronavirus jumped from Wuhan, China, to devastate the States, the United States can no longer afford to turn a blind eye to the next infectious outbreak, no matter where it occurs. But I also think empathy will play a role in how we respond to future health crises—which, in turn, has the potential to improve healthcare worldwide. As one of the greatest medical powers on the planet, the United States can tip the scales in favor of helping fight disease for everyone, not just because it helps Americans, but also because it is the right thing to do for the entire world.

Similarly, the pandemic also taught us how to work better together as an international medical community. During the outbreak, teams of researchers from all over the world have shared research and collaborated to help thwart COVID-19. While medicine has always had an international nexus, these connections are now more manifold and even stronger than ever before.

Silver Lining Medical Lesson #4: We Need to Rethink the Drug Supply Chain

During the early days of the outbreak, as hospitals scrambled to deal with patients with COVID-19, a different crisis was unfolding for doctors and the medical community at large: a critical shortage of prescription medications. The problem didn't arise because pharmacies in the United States were closed, but because manufacturing plants in China and other countries overseas had simply shut down—and most of our medications and medical equipment are manufactured abroad. In fact, China alone accounts for 90 percent of the United States' supply of antibiotics, ibuprofen, and hydrocortisone.[1]

The silver lining lesson here is that we can no longer afford to be dependent on other countries to produce our prescription drugs. What if the next outbreak—or natural disaster, political upheaval, or other disruptive crisis—lasts for a longer period of time, incapacitating foreign plant production for months instead of weeks? We can't enjoy the luxury of outsourcing our drug supply any longer. We should start manufacturing drugs domestically to avoid future shortage, which will only make our country more medically resilient.

Silver Lining Medical Lesson #5: Healthcare Workers Are Valuable, No Matter Their Age

I've always known that healthcare workers are heroes. Nearly everyone in my family is a doctor or a nurse, so I grew up seeing and hearing about the courage and self-sacrifice medical professionals show on a regular basis. The pandemic has now gifted the rest of the world with the respect I've had for my colleagues my entire life. That's a huge benefit, because healthcare workers have the potential to impact millions of lives, and the more respect they have, the easier it is for everyone to do their job.

But there's another silver lining lesson here when it comes to medical professionals. The pandemic has also shown us that healthcare workers of all ages are valuable assets in our new normal. During the initial outbreak, many states asked retired medical professionals to volunteer in hospitals and put their own lives on the line in order to counter an overwhelming staff shortage. In New York City alone, thousands of retired healthcare employees stepped up to answer the call.[2] If they hadn't, more lives certainly would have been lost. What this shows us is that people over sixty-five can have an imperative hands-on role in our society.

Silver Lining Medical Lesson #6: We Need to Rethink How We Treat Animals

Before the pandemic, very few people realized the role animals play in the spread of infectious disease. This included me—I was completely in the dark until I began talking with veterinarians and zoonotic experts. Now, thanks to the pandemic, more and more people are aware of what they've been warning us about for years: We need to rethink how we treat animals, especially those we use for food consumption, if we want to avoid the next outbreak.

Nearly every pandemic in human history has originated with animals, including the coronavirus.[3] Infectious diseases that spread from animals to humans are also responsible for a billion cases of illness around the planet every year.[4] The problem, however, isn't just live animal markets like those in Wuhan, China, where epidemiologists suspect the novel coronavirus may have originated. It's also traditional industrial farms where chickens, pigs, cows, and other commercial livestock are raised and slaughtered in oftentimes close or unhealthy conditions.[5]

I'm not suggesting we all become vegetarians. But the pandemic hopefully proves that it's time to prioritize raising livestock through organic or otherwise healthier methods in order to reduce the risk of zoonoses. It's also healthier, safer, and more humane for animals to be raised with more space and fewer antibiotics, not to mention healthier and safer for everyone who chooses to eat meat, as well.

Silver Lining Medical Lesson #7: Telemedicine Is a Good Thing

The pandemic didn't create telemedicine: Doctors have had the ability to see and treat patients virtually for years. But the outbreak accelerated the integration and use of telemedicine for millions of hospitals, medical clinics, and private practices. People who may have been hesitant to try the technology were forced to use it— many of them discovering that the virtual service can be just as effective and more convenient than in-person visits.

That telemedicine is often a good thing is a silver lining lesson for millions worldwide. Thanks to the pandemic, more patients now have—and know they have—access to quality healthcare. This is a game changer for many, especially those who live in rural or medically underserved areas, along with older people and any-one with disabilities who may have a difficult time making in-person appointments.

You probably don't need me to point out every single silver lining that has emerged from our new normal. There are many more sil-ver lining lessons that the pandemic has taught us, some of which may be difficult to behold at first blush, since they may look like disadvantages rather than benefits. But with every difficult lesson comes the opportunity to learn something valuable. Now it's up to all of us to use these valuable lessons to improve ourselves, not only as individuals but as communities and countries at large.

Epilogue

I'm not sure why I woke up at 1:03 A.M. that Friday, but I did. I had been sleeping soundly since 9:30 P.M. the night before, but maybe some intuitive sense or comic intervention caused me to sit up, get up, and go to the bathroom. Either way, one minute later, at 1:04 A.M., my phone started buzzing frantically by my bedside. A moment later, it was ringing. I picked up: The president of the United States had COVID-19.

Twenty minutes later, I was live and on-air by phone with the twenty-four-hour anchor team at ABC News. With the phone on speaker, I changed into a blouse and started putting on makeup and doing my hair. Another ten minutes later, I was powered up and on camera in my home studio delivering what would be the second of nearly a dozen different live reports on the president's diagnosis that I'd give over the next twenty-four hours.

That morning, after the president tweeted that he had tested positive for COVID-19, I was on the air from 1:30 A.M. to 3:15 A.M., breaking what would become not only the most significant health story but also the biggest story in the world. At 3:30 A.M., I went back to bed briefly for an hour before getting up again to prepare to be live on *Good Morning America,* WABC, *World News Tonight with David Muir, Nightline,* and other ABC shows. The next four days, as the virus exploded through the White House, I was live on-air for up to fourteen hours per day, just like I had been at the beginning of the coronavirus outbreak.

The Monday after the president's diagnosis, I had an hour-long phone call with my therapist—something I had made a priority after my ex-husband took his own life several years ago. But on that Monday, I didn't want to talk about my emotions, relationships, or what I could do to improve myself. I was so caught up in what I had experienced as a medical correspondent, a doctor, and an American citizen that I spent the first ten minutes of our sixty-minute call talking about President Trump's COVID-19 case.

That's when it came out: *I'm so sick of this virus. I'm sick of COVID-19.* I felt frustrated, hopeless, and worn down by the virus. I officially had pandemic fatigue.

I bet that you're sick of the virus, too. It's been months that we've been living like this, and the virus isn't going away. That's left a lot of people feeling frustrated and hopeless. And that's okay—that's a normal and natural response.

But while we're all sick of the virus, now is not the time to let your guard down. In fact, we have to remain more vigilant now than ever, as pandemic fatigue spreads and people start to get complacent. Case in point: President Trump.

The president's COVID-19 diagnosis proves what happens when you let your guard down. President Trump has gone on record many times saying he wouldn't wear a mask and has been televised not doing so in situations where it would have been recommended. He's also been televised not socially distancing in situations where it would have been recommended. The White House has been public about regularly testing the president and senior administration officials to help keep them safe. But testing, even at 1600 Pennsylvania Avenue, is not a prevention strategy—it's a surveillance and diagnostic approach. While the president may have escaped the virus for the first eight months of the outbreak, his behaviors eventually caught up with him, as the virus figured out a way into the most secure circle of power in the world. That's proof positive that no one can have a false sense of security or protection when it comes to this disease—not now and not another eight months from now.

The president's COVID-19 diagnosis also showed the world what doctors have known since the virus first appeared in Wuhan, China: COVID-19 can and does affect everyone. The virus doesn't need security clearance to penetrate the walls of the White House.

I want to be clear: These points have nothing to do with politics. While many people have politicized President Trump's diagnosis, for me, the story is medical and scientific. To quote *The New England Journal of Medicine* editorial on the United States' response to the pandemic, "Truth is neither liberal nor conservative."[1]

The need to politicize the president's COVID-19 diagnosis only underscores the degree of vitriolic emotions many have right now. As the pandemic has dragged on, it's become increasingly difficult to find calm in all the chaos. But we have to. And the way I've personally done so is to stick to what we know, which is the science, including the principles of infectious-disease control and the risk stratification outlined throughout this book.

Many businesses have reopened since the pandemic began and will continue to do so. More people are also traveling, eating out, and getting together with others in social situations—all good things. But this doesn't mean things are back to "normal." Just because more businesses are open and we're engaging in more everyday activities doesn't mean the virus packed up its bags and left the planet. It's still here, it's still a threat, and it will be a threat for years to come, even in the advent of an effective cure or vaccine.

I want to emphasize this point, because I think it's important not to develop a sense of false hope that any vaccine or vaccines, no matter how successful, will suddenly revert our world back to the way it was in 2019. At the time of this writing, 30 to 50 percent of Americans say they won't take a COVID-19 vaccine because they mistrust the process or have concerns over its safety and efficacy. That means many people won't have the protection a vaccine can provide.

What's more, doctors won't know for some time how long any vaccine will be able to protect those immunized against COVID-19. If the coronavirus is anything like the flu and mutates frequently, people may need to be inoculated every one to two years, which will pose real logistical challenges.

I'm not trying to be a killjoy. I think it's super important to remain cautiously optimistic that a vaccine can and will eventually put the pandemic in the world's rearview mirror. But in medicine as in life, while it's fine to look down the road, we have to keep our eyes focused on what's directly in front of us if we want to navigate our current world with any kind of precision and safety.

I realize that looking only at what's right in front of you can make it feel like there's no end in sight. I'd be lying if I told you that I haven't felt the same way at times, too. But that's why I've remained steadfast about focusing on the things that are important to me, like my family, my friends, my work, and a sense of self-care. I've also worked hard to try to manage my anxiety and remain grateful for everything in the world that is going right.

What's going right in your world? For one, you're alive—and that's no small feat. More Americans died during the first eight months of 2020 than during any other period of time since 1970, before aggressive antismoking and occupational-safety legislation was passed.[2] COVID-19 is now the third leading cause of death in the United States, beating out stroke, Alzheimer's, diabetes, and car crashes.

If you've been lucky enough to survive so far, that is certainly worth recognizing and celebrating. But it's not an indicator that you're immune or won't get infected at some point in the future.

I'm not trying to scare you—I just want to encourage you to remain realistic, vigilant, grateful, and hopeful.

Grateful and hopeful are what I want to leave you with, because there's a lot to be grateful and hopeful about these days. Pandemic or not, the world is still a wonderful, beautiful, and blessed place. Children are still being born, young people are still learning new things, couples are still getting married, and many of us are finding success, practicing the hobbies that make us happy, falling in love, and/or deepening our existing love with our family and friends.

There's no doubt about it: The virus has changed our world, transformed how we live, and upended our sense of normality. But I think it's important to remember that it hasn't overhauled who we are—and who we can be. In our new normal, you can still choose to be whatever you want to be. You can choose to be grateful, hopeful, and happy. You can choose to be kind, compassionate, and loving. And you can choose to be resilient. In short, you have the power to be your best self—no virus or pandemic will ever take that away.

Acknowledgments

I want to thank all who helped with this book, not necessarily in any order:

My ABC News family: It has been a privilege to work alongside the best team in network news during this historic time. The attention to detail, the concern for people's lives and feelings, and the vigor with which we have committed to this pandemic has made it an honor for me to be a part of such a team. This includes: James Goldston, Wendy Fisher, Marc Burstein, George Stephanopoulos, David Muir, Robin Roberts, Michael Strahan, Amy Robach, T. J. Holmes, JuJu Chang, Michael Corn, Simone Swink, Alberto Orso, Christine Brouwer, Mike Solmsen, Chris Dinan, Almin Karamehmedovic, Justin Dial, Catherine McKenzie and the entire *GMA3* team, my ABC News Radio family, Aaron Katersky, Eric Avram, Kerry Smith, Barbara Fedida, Debra O'Connell, Bill Ritter, Brian Teta, Terence Noonan, Steve Baker, John Green, David Sloan, Sony Salzman, Eden David, Brad Mielke, Katie DenDaas, and the operations team, along with our amazing directors, crew, makeup and hairstylists, and security team.

Eric Strauss: You are my right-hand person at ABC News, the most talented producer, the most diligent head of the ABC medical unit, and the greatest work partner. While you may speak softly and slowly, you get more accomplished than anyone I've ever met.

My coauthor, Sarah Toland: Working and writing with you is a personal and professional privilege. You are a beast on a deadline, a brilliant writer, and the best collaborator I could ask for.

My team at HarperCollins/William Morrow, including Lisa Sharkey: You always have your finger on the pulse of what people are interested in; and Matt Harper: You are a brilliant editor who is also just a really nice person.

My attorney, Bob Barnett: You are always calm, cheerful, and focused.

My medical practice, including my practice administrator, Carole Gittleman, and my medical assistant, Ana Olivera. We have worked together for more than fifteen years and are literally the three musketeers. Thank you for your commitment to our patients and for your friendship and support, both personally and professionally.

My patients: You inspire me every single day with your hunger for knowledge, your bravery, and your spirit. Your kind words of support mean the world to me.

My friends: Dr. Jennifer Haythe, Dr. Alice Kim, Dr. Patricia DeSalvo, Dr. Luis Diaz, Dr. Jeff Rapaport, and Dr. Adam Smith.

My family: my parents, Dorothy Garfein and Dr. Oscar Garfein; my brother, Dr. Evan Garfein; and my children, Alex and Chloe: I learn from you both every day, am inspired by you, and proud of the hearts and the minds you both have.

My favorite infectious disease experts: Dr. Todd Ellerin, vice chairman of medicine and director of infectious diseases at South Shore Health in Boston: Your medical insights and clinical expertise have been invaluable to me during this time. Your support means the world to me, before, during, and after COVID-19; Dr. Simone Wildes: You are a true role model to any girl who dreams of becoming a doctor; and Dr. Anthony Fauci: Knowing you and communicating directly with you throughout this (and other) historic viral outbreaks has been one of the most significant professional experiences in my medical career. Your elegance, along with your calm, warm, modest, and collegial personality, will always be remembered, and your service to the United States and the world's public health sphere has made a profound impact that will never be forgotten.

And to everyone, everywhere, who has been affected by or changed by COVID-19: You are not alone. I believe we will become more resilient as a result of COVID-19, we will learn from our mistakes, we will celebrate our triumphs, and we will be more prepared for the next pandemic. We will get through this because we are all in this together.

Notes

CHAPTER 1: BODY

1 Christopher H. Herbst, Reem F. Alsukait, Mohammed Alluhidan, Nahar Alazemi, and Meera Shekar, "Individuals with Obesity and COVID-19: A Global . . . ," Wiley Online Library, https://online library.wiley.com/doi/full/10.1111/obr.13128, accessed August 26, 2020.

2 Christopher M. Petrill, Simon A. Jones, Jie Yang, Harish Rajago-palan, Luke O'Donnell, Yelena Chernyak, Katie A. Tobin, Robert J. Cerfolio, Fritz Francois, and Leora I. Horowitz, "Largest US Study of COVID-19: Obesity Single Biggest Chronic Factor," *Physician's Weekly,* April 14, 2020.

3 Roni Caryn Rabin, "Obesity Linked to Severe Coronavirus Disease, Especially for Younger Patients," *New York Times,* April 16, 2020.

4 David C. W. Lau, "Practical Approaches to the Treatment of Obesity," Julia McFarlane Diabetes Research Centre, https://www .accrockies.com/downloads/slides/2012/1_Sunday/Sunday_04 _Lau_Obesity_Rx.pdf, March 11, 2012.

5 "COVID-19 Study Shows More Than 4 Times In-Hospital Mortality Rate and Increased Length of Stay for Patients with Diabetes and Hyperglycemia," Business Wire, April 17, 2020.

6 Sara Rigby, "Coronavirus: High Blood Pressure Could Double Risk of Death," *BBC Science Focus Magazine,* June 5, 2020.

7   "High Blood Pressure Linked to Increased Risk of Dying from COVID-19," European Society of Cardiology, June 5, 2020.

8   "Facts About Hypertension," Centers for Disease Control and Prevention, September 8, 2020.

9   "Million Hearts® Undiagnosed Hypertension," Centers for Disease Control and Prevention, Division for Heart Disease and Stroke Prevention, November 8, 2019.

10 Brunilda Nazario, "Coronavirus and High Blood Pressure: What's the Link?" WebMD, September 23, 2020.

11 Bruce Goldman, "High Blood Pressure Drugs Don't Increase COVID-19 Risk, Stanford Study Finds," Scope 10k (blog), Stanford Medicine, July 14, 2020.

12 Emily Ihara, Health Policy Institute, Georgetown University, February 13, 2019.

13 Roengrudee Patanavich and Stanton A. Glantz, "Smoking Is Associated with COVID-19 Progression: A Meta-Analysis," *Nicotine & Tobacco Research* 22, no. 9 (September 2020): 1653–56.

14 Erin Digitale, "Vaping Linked to COVID-19 Risk in Teens and Young Adults," Stanford Medicine News Center, Stanford Medicine, August 11, 2020.

15 Serena Gordon, "Vaping-Related Lung Injuries Still Happening— And May Look Like COVID-19," *U.S. News & World Report,* June 30, 2020.

16 "Chronic Diseases in America," Centers for Disease Control and Prevention, October 23, 2019.

CHAPTER 2: MIND

1   Joel Achenbach, "Coronavirus Is Harming the Mental Health of Tens of Millions of People in U.S., New Poll Finds," *Washington Post,* April 2, 2020.

2   William Wan, "The Coronavirus Pandemic Is Pushing America into a Mental Health Crisis," *Washington Post,* May 12, 2020.

3   James Hamblin, "Is Everyone Depressed?" *The Atlantic,* May 22, 2020.

4   "Substantial Investment Needed to Avert Mental Health Crisis," World Health Organization, May 14, 2020.

5   Robin Wright, "How Loneliness from Coronavirus Isolation Takes Its Toll," *The New Yorker,* March 23, 2020.

6 Daisuke Nishi, Shigenobu Kanba, and Tadafumi Kato, "Mental Health Issues Associated with COVID-19 Outbreak," virtual issue, *Psychiatry and Clinical Neurosciences,* Wiley Online Library, April 20, 2020.

7 Wright, "Loneliness from Coronavirus Isolation."

8 "Loneliness and Social Isolation Linked to Serious Health Conditions," Centers for Disease Control and Prevention, May 26, 2020.

9 "The 'Loneliness Epidemic,'" U.S. Health Resources & Services Administration, January 10, 2019.

10 "The Rise in Alcohol & Drug Relapses from Coronavirus," Banyan Treatment Centers, June 15, 2020.

11 Kristen Monaco, "Mental Health Challenges After COVID-19 Recovery," Medical News and Free CME Online, MedpageToday, May 18, 2020.

12 Lisa L. Colangelo, "'Not Alone': Mental Health Experts Help Patients Cope After COVID-19," *Newsday,* June 29, 2020.

13 Melinda Smith, Lawrence Robinson, and Jeanne Segal, "Coping with Grief and Loss," HelpGuide, September 2020.

14 Judith Rodin, *The Resilience Dividend: Being Strong in a World Where Things Go Wrong* (New York: PublicAffairs, 2014).

CHAPTER 3: HEALTHCARE

1 William Booth, Aaron Gregg, and Isaac Stanley-Becker, "Americans Warned of 'Pearl Harbor Moment' as Trump Tells Parts of the Nation to Brace for 'Peak,'" *Washington Post,* April 6, 2020.

2 Alejandro de la Garza, "Emergency Room Visits Plunge During COVID-19 Pandemic," *Time,* June 4, 2020.

3 Will Stone and Elly Yu, "Empty ERs Worry Doctors as Heart Attack and Stroke Patients Delay Care," *U.S. News & World Report,* May 8, 2020.

4 Alexandra Galante, "After Man, 38, Dies of Heart Attack, Wife Shares Urgent Message: 'Go to the ER,'" TODAY.com, June 16, 2020.

5 Kathleen P. Hartnett, Aaron Kite-Powell, Jourdan DeVies, Michael A. Coletta, Tegan K. Boehmer, Jennifer Adjemian, and Adi V. Gundlapalli, "Impact of the COVID-19 Pandemic on Emergency

Department Visits—United States, January 1, 2019–May 30, 2020," Centers for Disease Control and Prevention, June 11, 2020.

6 Steven H. Woolf, Derek A. Chapman, and Roy T. Sabo, "Excess Deaths from COVID-19 and Other Causes, March–April 2020," *JAMA,* August 4, 2020.

7 "More People Are Dying During the Pandemic—And Not Just from COVID-19," American Heart Association, June 16, 2020.

8 Greg Jaffe and Amy Brittain, "Obama: 'We Can't Give in to Hysteria or Fear' of Ebola," *Washington Post,* October 18, 2014.

9 Stephanie Evans, Emily Agnew, Emilia Vynnycky, and Julie V. Robotham, "The Impact of Testing and Infection Prevention and Control Strategies on Within-Hospital Transmission Dynamics of COVID-19 in English Hospitals," *MedRxiv,* May 20, 2020.

10 Rich Daly, "Preventable ED Use Costs $8.3 Billion Annually: Analysis," Healthcare Financial Management Association, February 11, 2019.

11 Lori Uscher-Pines, Jesse Pines, Arthur Kellermann, Emily Gillen, and Ateev Mehrotra, "Deciding to Visit the Emergency Department for Non-Urgent Conditions: A Systematic Review of the Literature," September 5, 2014.

12 Oleg Bestsennyy, Greg Gilbert, Alex Harris, and Jennifer Rost, "Telehealth: A Quarter-Trillion-Dollar Post-COVID-19 Reality?" McKinsey & Company, June 1, 2020.

13 Ibid.

14 Kimberly Lankford, "4 Ways Telehealth Can Save You Money," *U.S. News & World Report,* April 6, 2020.

15 Ana Blasco, Montserrat Carmona, Ignacio Fernández-Lozano, Carlos H. Salvador, Mario Pascual, Pilar G. Sagredo, Roberto Somolinos, et al. "Evaluation of a Telemedicine Service for the Secondary Prevention of Coronary Artery Disease," *Journal of Cardiopulmonary Rehabilitation and Prevention* 32, no. 1 (2012): 25–31.

16 Mary Van Beusekom, "In Pandemic, Many Seeing Upsides to Telemedicine," Center for Infectious Disease Research and Policy, University of Minnesota, May 21, 2020.

CHAPTER 4: FOOD

1   Junxiu Liu, Colin D. Rehm, Renata Micha, and Dariush Mozaffarian, "Quality of Meals Consumed by US Adults at Full-Service and Fast-Food Restaurants, 2003–2016: Persistent Low Quality and Widening Disparities," *The Journal of Nutrition* 150, no. 4 (2020): 873–83.

2   Megan Meyer, "2020 Food and Health Survey," Food Insight, International Food Information Council, July 7, 2020.

3   Ibid.

4   Anagha Srikanth, "Americans Are Gaining Weight and Buying More Fitness Equipment in Quarantine, But Are They Using It?" The Hill, July 6, 2020.

5   Rajeshni Naidu-Ghelani, "Comfort Food: Women More Likely to Admit to Overeating, Under Exercising amid COVID-19," Ipsos, May 28, 2020.

6   Josie Delap, "Why Sourdough Went Viral," *The Economist,* August 4, 2020.

7   Rasha Ali, "New Quarantine Cooking Trend Alert: Get Ready to Dig into a Bowl of Pancake Cereal," *USA Today,* May 16, 2020.

8   Kim Severson, "7 Ways the Pandemic Has Changed How We Shop for Food," *New York Times,* September 8, 2020.

9   Debbie Koenig, "Quarantine Weight Gain Not a Joking Matter," WebMD, May 21, 2020.

10 Srikanth, "Americans Are Gaining Weight and Buying More Fitness Equipment in Quarantine."

11 Sarah Maslin Nir, "Tailors Know New Yorkers' Pandemic Secret: 'Everybody Got Fat!'" *New York Times,* July 25, 2020.

12 Alexandra Ashbrook, "Nearly 60 Percent Increase in Older Adult Food Insecurity During COVID-19: Federal Action on SNAP Needed Now," Food Research & Action Center, July 31, 2020.

13 Gianna Melillo, "Hyperglycemia Is an Independent Risk Factor of COVID-19 Mortality," *The American Journal of Managed Care,* July 18, 2020.

14 E. J. Mundell, "COVID-19 May Spike Blood Sugar, Raising Death Risk," WebMD, July 13, 2020.

15 "COVID-19 and Diabetes," International Diabetes Federation, August 27, 2020.

16 "How Much Sugar Is Too Much?" American Heart Association, n.d.

17 Sara Chodosh, "Sorry, Keto Fans, You're Probably Not in Ketosis," *Popular Science,* June 8, 2020.

18 Adrian R. Martineau and Nita G. Forouhi, "Vitamin D for COVID-19: A Case to Answer?" *The Lancet Diabetes & Endocrinology* 8, no. 9 (2020): 735–36.

19 "Office of Dietary Supplements—Vitamin D," NIH Office of Dietary Supplements, U.S. Department of Health and Human Services, September 11, 2020.

20 Megan Meyer, "COVID-19 Pandemic Transforms the Way We Shop, Eat and Think About Food, According to IFIC's 2020 Food & Health Survey," Food Insight, International Food Information Council.

21 "Study Suggests Home Cooking Is a Main Ingredient in Healthier Diet," Center for a Livable Future, Johns Hopkins Bloomberg School of Public Health, November 17, 2014.

22 Hans Taparia, "How Covid-19 Is Making Millions of Americans Healthier," *New York Times,* April 18, 2020.

23 Severson, "7 Ways the Pandemic Has Changed How We Shop for Food."

24 Mary Knight, "How Much Money Do You Save by Cooking at Home?" Wellio, July 10, 2018.

25 "Cooking at Home Tonight? It's Likely Cheaper and Healthier, Study Finds," ScienceDaily, March 14, 2017.

26 "Happy Couples: How to Keep Your Relationship Healthy," American Psychological Association, January 1, 2020.

27 Steven Reinberg, "Typical Restaurant Meal Loaded with Fats, Salt, Calories: Studies," WebMD, n.d.

28 "Meals at 92 Percent of Dining Establishments Tip the Scales," ScienceDaily, January 20, 2016.

CHAPTER 5: EXERCISE

1 Jacob Meyer, Cillian McDowell, Jeni Lansing, Cassandra Brower, Lee Smith, Mark Tully, and Matthew Herring, "Changes in Physical Activity and Sedentary Behaviour Due to the COVID-19 Outbreak and Associations with Mental Health in 3,052 US Adults," *Cambridge Open Engage,* 2020.

2 Jamie Ducharme, "COVID-19 Is Making Americans Even More Sedentary: The Effects Could Be Long-Lasting," May 12, 2020.

3 Ibid.

4 "Survey Reveals Gyms Will Never Be the Same After Coronavirus," LIFEAID Beverage Co. Blog, June 27, 2020.

5 Jade Scipioni, "59% of Americans Don't Plan to Renew Their Gym Memberships After Covid-19 Pandemic: Survey," CNBC.com, July 23, 2020.

6 "Survey Reveals Gyms Will Never Be the Same."

7 "COVID-19: Exercise May Help Prevent Deadly Complication," UVA Health Newsroom, University of Virginia Health System, April 15, 2020.

8 University of Bath, "Regular Exercise Benefits Immunity—Even in Isolation," ScienceDaily.

9 "Exercise Is an All-Natural Treatment to Fight Depression," Harvard Health Publishing, Harvard Medical School, July 2013.

10 "Exercise for Stress and Anxiety," Anxiety and Depression Association of America.

11 Rachel P. Tillage, Genevieve E. Wilson, L. Cameron Liles, Philip V. Holmes, and David Weinshenker, "Chronic Environmental or Genetic Elevation of Galanin in Noradrenergic Neurons Confers Stress Resilience in Mice," *Journal of Neuroscience* 40, no. 39 (2020): 7464–74.

12 Lawrence Robinson, Jeanne Segal, and Melinda Smith, "The Mental Health Benefits of Exercise," HelpGuide, June 2019.

13 ABCNews, "Ohio Man Builds Exercise Equipment from Timber After Gym Shuts Down over Coronavirus," YouTube.com, April 8, 2020.

14 John Hanc, "Keeping Clients Fit During the Pandemic by Going Virtual," *New York Times,* May 26, 2020.

CHAPTER 6: SLEEP

1 "Sleep Habits Post Lockdown in the U.S.," Sleep Standards, May 2020.

2 Natana Raj, "Sleep Aids: Technologies and Global Markets," BCC Research, April 2020.

3 "Sleep Habits Post Lockdown in the U.S."

4 Ibid.

5 Ibid.

6 Dan Hurley, "Sleep Neurologists Call It 'COVID-Somnia'—Increased Sleep Disturbances Linked to the Pandemic," *Neurology Today* 20, no. 13 (2020).

7 James M. Lang, "Kids Are Spending More Hours on Screens Than Ever: Should Parents Worry?" *Fast Company,* July 20, 2020.

8 Kelli Miller, "COVID and Sleep: Sweet Dreams Aren't Made of This," WebMD, May 27, 2020.

9 Eric J. Olson, "Can Lack of Sleep Make You Sick?" Mayo Clinic, Mayo Foundation for Medical Education and Research, November 28, 2018.

10 Samir Deshpande and Walter Reed, "A Full Night's Sleep Could Be the Best Defense Against COVID-19," Health.mil, Military Health System, March 23, 2020.

11 Elizabeth Fernandez, "Sleep Affects Potency of Vaccines," University of California San Francisco, August 1, 2012.

12 Chun Shing Kwok, Evangelos Kontopantelis, George Kuligowski, Matthew Gray, Alan Muhyaldeen, Christopher P. Gale, George M. Peat, et al. "Self-Reported Sleep Duration and Quality and Cardiovascular Disease and Mortality: A Dose-Response Meta-Analysis," *Journal of the American Heart Association* 7, no. 15 (2018).

13 "What Temperature Should Your Bedroom Be?" Sleep Foundation, July 28, 2020.

14 Julie Corliss, "Mindfulness Meditation Helps Fight Insomnia, Improves Sleep," Harvard Health Blog, Harvard Health Publishing, June 15, 2020.

15 Deirdre Barrett, "The 'Committee of Sleep': A Study of Dream Incubation for Problem Solving," *Dreaming* 3, no. 2 (1993): 115–22.

16 "COVID-19 TV Habits Suggest the Days Are Blurring Together," Comcast Corporation, May 6, 2020.

17 Ibid.

18 "Coronavirus Pandemic and Americans Sleep (2020 Data)," Sleep Standards, June 11, 2020.

19 "COVID-19 TV Habits."

20   "Long-Term Ambien Use and Severe Addiction," American Addiction Centers, September 30, 2019.

CHAPTER 7: HEALTH FEARS

1   "Pedestrian Fatalities on Interstate Highways, United States, 1993–2012," AAA Foundation for Traffic Safety, September 14, 2012.
2   Annelieke M. Roest, Elisabeth J. Martens, Peter De Jonge, and Johan Denollet, "Anxiety and Risk of Incident Coronary Heart Disease: A Meta-Analysis," *Journal of the American College of Cardiology* 56, no. 1 (2010): 38–46.
3   Allison Aubrey, Laurel Wamsley, and Carmel Wroth, "From Camping to Dining Out: Here's How Experts Rate the Risks of 14 Summer Activities," NPR, May 23, 2020.
4   "Always Worried About Your Health? You May Be Dealing with Health Anxiety Disorder," Harvard Health Publishing, Harvard Medical School, September 2018.
5   University of Bath, "Lockdown Study Reports Surge in Health Anxieties: New Research into People's Coping Strategies Faced with COVID-19 Highlights the Mental Health Toll for Those Shielding," ScienceDaily, August 4, 2020.
6   Amy Gunia, "'I Don't Think We Should Ever Shake Hands Again': Dr. Fauci Says Coronavirus Should Change Some Behaviors for Good," *Time,* April 9, 2020.
7   Clare Lally, "Child and Adolescent Mental Health During COVID-19," POST, UK Parliament, July 14, 2020.
8   "Signs You May Be a Hypochondriac," Center for Treatment of Anxiety and Mood Disorders, June 15, 2020.
9   Ken Goodman, "Health Anxiety: What It Is and How to Beat It," Anxiety and Depression Association of America, June 22, 2020.
10   Honor Whiteman, "Cognitive Behavioral Therapy 'Effective' for Health Anxiety," *Medical News Today,* October 19, 2013.
11   Molly Jong-Fast, "Why Are So Many Baby Boomers in Denial Over the Coronavirus?" *Vogue,* March 13, 2020.
12   "United States COVID-19 Cases and Deaths by State," Centers for Disease Control and Prevention, n.d.
13   "What Are the Odds of Dying From . . . ," National Safety Council, n.d.

14   "Fifty Quotations by Ralph Waldo Emerson," Walden Woods Project, Thoreau Institute at Walden Woods, n.d.

15   Isabel Reche, Gaetano D'Orta, Natalie Mladenov, Danielle M. Winget, and Curtis A. Suttle, "Deposition Rates of Viruses and Bacteria Above the Atmospheric Boundary Layer," *The ISME Journal* 12, no. 4 (2018): 1154–62.

16   Eniola Kasim, "The Wonderful World of Virology," Institute for Public Health (blog), July 9, 2019.

17   "CDC Updates COVID-19 Transmission Webpage to Clarify Information About Types of Spread," CDC Newsroom, Centers for Disease Control and Prevention, May 22, 2020.

18   "How COVID-19 Spreads," Centers for Disease Control and Prevention, September 21, 2020.

19   "Cleaning and Disinfection for Households," Centers for Disease Control and Prevention, July 10, 2020.

20   Terry Gross, "'The Beautiful Cure' Reveals the 'Profound' Power of the Immune System," *Fresh Air,* NPR, November 26, 2018.

21   Suzanne C. Segerstrom and Sandra E. Sephton, "Optimistic Expectancies and Cell-Mediated Immunity," *Psychological Science* 21, no. 3 (2010): 448–55.

22   Natalie B. Compton, "People Are Wearing Hazmat Suits on Planes: But Should They?" *Washington Post,* May 25, 2020.

23   Darwin Malicdem, "Your Favorite Bleach Could Produce Dangerous Indoor Air Pollutants," Medical Daily, October 3, 2019.

24   "Cleaning Supplies and Your Health," EWG, n.d.

CHAPTER 8: MEDICAL NEWS

1   "Remarks by President Trump, Vice President Pence, and Members of the Coronavirus Task Force in Press Briefing," White House.gov, April 3, 2020.

2   Sonal Desai, "On My Mind: They Blinded Us from Science," Franklin Templeton Investments, July 29, 2020.

3   Mark Jurkowitz and Amy Mitchell, "Coronavirus Stories Cited as Made-Up News Include Claims About Risks, Details of Virus," Pew Research Center's Journalism Project, August 18, 2020.

4   Md Saiful Islam, Tonmoy Sarkar, Sazzad Hossain Khan, Abu-

Hena Mostofa Kamal, S. M. Murshid Hasan, Alamgir Kabir, Dalia Yeasmin, et al. "COVID-19–Related Infodemic and Its Impact on Public Health: A Global Social Media Analysis," *The American Journal of Tropical Medicine and Hygiene* 103, no. 4 (2020): 1621–29.

5 Tedros Adhanom Ghebreyesus, "Munich Security Conference," World Health Organization, February 15, 2020.

6 "1st WHO Infodemiology Conference," World Health Organization, July 16, 2020.

7 Mark Jurkowitz, Amy Mitchell, J. Baxter Oliphant, and Elisa Shearer, "Three Months In, Many Americans See Exaggeration, Conspiracy Theories and Partisanship in COVID-19 News," Pew Research Center's Journalism Project, September 18, 2020.

8 Sarah Kreps and Douglas Kriner, "Good News and Bad News About COVID-19 Misinformation," *Scientific American,* June 10, 2020.

9 Jurkowitz et al., "Three Months In."

10 Ryan Broderick, "'I'm Not an Epidemiologist But . . .': The Rise of the Coronavirus Influencers," BuzzFeed News, March 18, 2020.

11 Julian E. Barnes and David E. Sanger, "Russian Intelligence Agencies Push Disinformation on Pandemic," *New York Times,* July 28, 2020.

12 Jennifer Rankin, "EU Says China Behind 'Huge Wave' of Covid-19 Disinformation," *Guardian,* June 10, 2020.

13 Monica Gandhi and George W. Rutherford, "Facial Masking for Covid-19—Potential for 'Variolation' as We Await a Vaccine," *The New England Journal of Medicine,* September 8, 2020.

14 B. Blocken, F. Malizia, T. van Druenen, and T. Marchal, "Towards Aerodynamically Equivalent COVID-19 1.5m Social Distancing for Walking and Running," 2020.

15 Sigal Samuel, "Why You're Unlikely to Get the Coronavirus from Runners or Cyclists," VOX, August 13, 2020.

16 Eric Niiler, "Are Running or Cycling Actually Risks for Spreading Covid-19?" *Wired,* April 14, 2020.

17 Heena Sahni and Hunny Sharma, "Role of Social Media During the COVID-19 Pandemic: Beneficial, Destructive, or Reconstructive?" *International Journal of Academic Medicine* 6, no. 2 (June 29, 2020): 70–75.

18 Kreps and Kriner, "Good News and Bad News About COVID-19 Misinformation."

19 Emma Graham-Harrison and Alex Hern, "Facebook Funnelling Readers Towards Covid Misinformation—Study," *Guardian,* August 19, 2020.

20 Katie Paul and Munsif Vengattil, "Facebook Removed Seven Million Posts in Second Quarter for False Coronavirus Information," Thomson Reuters, August 11, 2020.

21 "How Facebook Can Flatten the Curve of the Coronavirus Infodemic," Avaaz, April 15, 2020.

22 Amy Mitchell, Galen Stocking, and Katerina Eva Matsa, "Some Readers Willing to Dig into Long-Form News on Cellphones," Pew Research Center's Journalism Project, May 30, 2020.

23 E. J. Mundell, " 'COVID Toe' Probably Not Caused by COVID-19," WebMD, June 25, 2020.

24 Kim Schive, "Will Gargling Wash the Virus Away?" MIT Medical, April 13, 2020.

CHAPTER 9: FAMILY AND FRIENDS

1 "Older Adults and COVID-19," Centers for Disease Control and Prevention, September 11, 2020.

2 "COVID-19 Hospitalization and Death by Age," Centers for Disease Control and Prevention, September 11, 2020.

3 "Children's Role in Spread of Virus Bigger Than Thought," *Harvard Gazette,* August 20, 2020.

4 Robert L. DeBiasi and Meghan Delaney, "Symptomatic and Asymptomatic Viral Shedding in Pediatric Patients Infected with Severe Acute Respiratory Syndrome Coronavirus 2 (SARS-CoV-2): Under the Surface," *JAMA Pediatrics,* August 28, 2020.

5 "Health Department-Reported Cases of Multisystem Inflammatory Syndrome in Children (MIS-C) in the United States," Centers for Disease Control and Prevention, September 18, 2020.

6 "CDC Childhood Injury Report," Centers for Disease Control and Prevention, February 6, 2019.

7 "As Pandemic Drags On, Relationships Are Getting More Serious," Ipsos, August 4, 2020.

8　Andy Fies, "Surge in Divorces Anticipated in Wake of COVID-19 Quarantine," ABCNews, April 17, 2020.

9　"As Pandemic Drags On, Relationships."

10　Ibid.

11　"What to Do If Your Pet Tests Positive for the Virus That Causes COVID-19," Centers for Disease Control and Prevention, September 10, 2020.

12　Ibid.

CHAPTER 10: PUBLIC PLACES

1　Tim Heffernan, "Can HEPA Air Purifiers Capture the Coronavirus?" *New York Times,* July 9, 2020.

2　"How HEPA Filters Have Been Purifying Cabin Air Since the 1990s," American Airlines Newsroom, June 26, 2020.

3　Arnold Barnett, "Covid-19 Risk Among Airline Passengers: Should the Middle Seat Stay Empty?" *MedRxiv,* August 2, 2020.

4　Ibid.

5　Ibid.

6　Jessica Craig, "Can Air Conditioners Spread COVID-19?" NPR, August 15, 2020.

7　"Air Conditioning Risks?" MIT Medical, June 23, 2020.

8　"Q&A: Ventilation and Air Conditioning in Public Spaces and Buildings and COVID-19," World Health Organization, July 29, 2020.

9　Choe Sang-Hun, "South Korea Warns of Another Covid-19 Outbreak Tied to a Church," *New York Times,* August 16, 2020.

10　Allison James, Lesli Eagle, Cassandra Phillips, Stephen Hedges, Cathie Bodenhamer, Robin Brown, J. Gary Wheeler, and Hannah Kirking, "High COVID-19 Attack Rate Among Attendees at Events at a Church—Arkansas, March 2020," Centers for Disease Control and Prevention, May 21, 2020.

11　Kate Conger, Jack Healy, and Lucy Tompkins, "Churches Were Eager to Reopen: Now They Are Confronting Coronavirus Cases," *New York Times,* July 8, 2020.

12　Megan Hart, "Sheboygan County Outbreak Highlights Risks of Reopening Church During Pandemic," Wisconsin Public Radio, June 17, 2020.

13   Allison Aubrey, Laurel Wamsley, and Carmel Wroth, "From Camping to Dining Out: Here's How Experts Rate the Risks of 14 Summer Activities," WBUR News, May 23, 2020.

CHAPTER 11: SILVER LININGS
1   Ana Swanson, "Coronavirus Spurs U.S. Efforts to End China's Chokehold on Drugs," *New York Times,* March 11, 2020.
2   "Retired Doctors and Nurses Don Scrubs Again in Coronavirus Fight," *U.S. News & World Report,* March 27, 2020.
3   Charlie Campbell, "Don't Blame China: The Next Pandemic Could Come from Anywhere," *Time,* March 10, 2020.
4   Christian Walzer, "The COVID-19 Pandemic Has Introduced Us to a New Word: Zoonosis (Op-Ed)," LiveScience, April 1, 2020.
5   Ananya Mandal, "Could the Next Pandemic Be 100 Times Worse Than COVID-19?" News Medical Life Sciences, June 2, 2020.

EPILOGUE
1   https://www.nejm.org/doi/full/10.1056/NEJMe2029812.
2   https://www.scientificamerican.com/article/covid-19-is-now-the -third-leading-cause-of-death-in-the-u-s1/.

About the Authors

Dr. Jennifer Ashton is the chief medical correspondent of ABC News, including *Good Morning America, World News Tonight with David Muir, Nightline,* and *GMA3: What You Need to Know.* Since joining ABC in 2012, Ashton has reported on a range of medical topics including the maternal mortality crisis, mental illness and suicide, and heart disease. At the onset of the 2020 coronavirus outbreak, Ashton appeared as the featured medical correspondent on ABC News's *Pandemic: What You Need to Know* and has covered the outbreak extensively for the network since then, talking regularly with the world's leading infectious-disease doctors. Ashton has met with the CDC director, visited the National Institutes of Health's vaccine development lab with Dr. Anthony Fauci, and met with members of the Coronavirus Task Force at the White House. In 2009, she received the Alfred I. duPont-Columbia Award for Excellence in Journalism for her work in television medical reporting.

Dr. Ashton is a graduate of Columbia College, Columbia University, and Columbia Medical School. She completed her residency training in obstetrics and gynecology and received a Master of Science degree in nutrition from Columbia University. She is board-certified in OB-GYN and obesity medicine and maintains a private clinical practice in New Jersey. The author of five other books, Ashton lives in New York City with her two children.

Sarah Toland is the coauthor of several bestselling books, including the *New York Times* bestselling *Strong Is the New Beautiful* with Lindsey Vonn. A former editor for *Men's Journal, Prevention,* and other national magazines, Toland has also written for the *New York Times, Sports Illustrated*, and a handful of other eminent publications. Toland lives in New York City.